Ventilation/blood flow and gas exchange

To Hermann Rahn

Ventilation/blood flow
and gas exchange

John B. West M D (Adelaide) Ph D (London)

*Professor of Medicine and Bioengineering,
School of Medicine, University of California at
San Diego, La Jolla, California.
(Formerly, Reader, Department of Medicine,
Postgraduate Medical School and Consultant
Clinical Respiratory Physiologist, Hammersmith
Hospital, London)*

Second edition
Second printing

Blackwell Scientific Publications
Oxford and Edinburgh

ISBN 0 632 07030 7

First published December 1965
Reprinted May 1967
Second edition 1970
Reprinted 1971

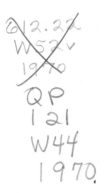
Distributed in the U.S.A by
F. A. Davis Company, 1915 Arch Street,
Philadelphia, Pennsylvania

Printed in Great Britain by
Lowe & Brydone (Printers) Ltd, London,
and bound by
The Kemp Hall Bindery, Oxford

Contents

Preface to First Edition

This monograph arose out of lectures given at the Postgraduate Medical School, and particularly three invited lectures at the Westminster Hospital Medical School in the autumn of 1964. Presenting clinical respiratory physiology today is not easy because the advances have been so fast in the last 20 years that many doctors have elected to wait until the subject settles down and the terminology sorts itself out. Thus some degree of immunity has often been developed.

However the relations between ventilation, blood flow and gas exchange are of great practical importance because ventilation-perfusion ratio inequality is the chief cause of hypoxaemia in the medical wards. The subject is not an easy one and any serious attempt to understand it must take advantage of the oxygen-carbon dioxide diagram which has proved to be such a powerful tool. This monograph begins at an elementary level and aims to bridge the gap between the simple review article and the original papers on ventilation-perfusion ratio inequality. This restricted field has been deliberately chosen because it is the most important aspect of gas exchange and the most difficult to understand. It is hoped that this monograph will be a painless introduction to the ventilation-perfusion ratio for the resident and consultant physician who are interested in lung function as well as for the physiologist.

To this end, equations have been omitted almost entirely from the text because they invariably provoke resistance in many people. However there are a great many diagrams and graphs which contain the same ingredients in a more palatable form. For the same reason, the text contains relatively few references because these distract the reader, although those who talk the $\dot{V}_A/\dot{Q}$ language will immediately realize that this book contains virtually nothing that is new.

Many colleagues and friends have read the manuscript and

suggested improvements. These include Dr G.Brandi, Dr E.J.M. Campbell, Dr J.E.Cotes, Dr L.E.Farhi, Dr C.M.Fletcher, Dr B.E. Heard, Dr M.C.F.Pain, Dr H.Rahn and Dr M.K.Sykes. I wish to express my gratitude to all these. The experimental work described in chapter 2 was done in conjunction with Dr C.T.Dollery, Dr P.Hugh-Jones and others, and it owes much to the constant support of Sir John McMichael F.R.S., and to Mr D.D.Vonberg and the M.R.C. Cyclotron Unit for facilities. The work was supported by the Medical Research Council.

Preface to Second Edition

On the assumption that the success of this little monograph is in large measure due to its brevity, few additions have been made to the second edition. Most of the changes are in Chapter 2 which has been brought up-to-date. The author is grateful to the many readers who have queried various points and hopes that these dialogues will continue.

Introduction

This small monograph attempts to answer the question: how does inequality of blood flow and ventilation in the lung interfere with gas exchange, that is the ability of the lung to take up oxygen and put out carbon dioxide. Because this mechanism is the chief cause of arterial hypoxaemia in the medical wards, the question is important to the physician as well as to the physiologist. The problem is approached by first looking at the normal lung because recent work has shown that its inequality of blood flow and ventilation follow a simple topographical pattern. For this reason, the regional differences of gas exchange can be set out like a map, and although the abnormal lung is not so amenable, the same principles apply. Overall gas exchange is approached through the oxygen-carbon dioxide diagram because in a simple form this is an invaluable tool in this field. Just as a diagram is useful in understanding acid-base balance in the body, so the oxygen-carbon dioxide diagram allows the impairment of gas exchange in the diseased lung to be easily grasped.

The plan of the book is as follows. Chapter 1 takes a bird's eye view of the movement of oxygen from the atmosphere to the blood by the lung and thus introduces the various causes of arterial hypoxaemia. Chapter 2 examines the distribution of blood flow and ventilation in the normal upright lung and derives the pattern of ventilation-perfusion ratio inequality. Chapter 3 takes this pattern of ventilation-perfusion ratio inequality and by means of the oxygen-carbon dioxide diagram, deduces differences in regional gas exchange. In chapter 4, the resulting impairment of overall gas transfer is examined, and the normal lung is compared with the abnormal lung where the pattern is less orderly but the effects are far more dramatic. Chapter 5 deals with ways of measuring ventilation-perfusion ratio inequality, and shows how this mechanism can be distinguished from other causes of arterial hypoxaemia.

Chapter 1

Oxygen transport from air to tissues

The lung unit

The prime function of the lung is to exchange gas or, in other words, to arterialize venous blood. A logical starting point for a discussion of lung physiology is therefore the alveolar membrane through which the gas exchange occurs. This is shown in figure 1 as a single thin line. In practice, the gas-blood interface is some 100 square metres in area with a mean thickness of less than 1 micron. If its thickness were increased to 1 cm and its relative dimensions remained the same, the interface would cover the whole of Wales (or Connecticut) so that its shape is well suited to its gas-exchanging function.

Air is brought to one side of the interface and blood to the other. Figure 1 shows the alveolar gas volume, that is the gas which is actively engaged in exchanging oxygen and carbon dioxide. This space is connected to the outside air by a system of conducting airways, the bronchi and bronchioles. This volume is called the anatomic dead space because the gas within does not take part in gas exchange. On the other side of the alveolar membrane is the pulmonary capillary fed by a pulmonary arteriole and draining into a venule. As blood passes along the capillary, it takes up oxygen and gives off carbon dioxide.

This then is the unit of lung function analogous to the nephron, for example, which is the functional unit of the kidney. Two features of the lung unit may be emphasised at this stage. One is its symmetry, that is the fact that gas and blood are equally important in its function. This simple fact is not always appreciated in that sometimes the lung is regarded chiefly as a pump which moves air in and out of the chest. It certainly does this, but only as a means to an end which is gas exchange, and for this prime function gas and blood are equally important.

The other feature of the lung unit is its simplicity. Compare it, for example, with the nephron with its glomerulus, proximal convuluted tubule, descending and ascending loops of Henle, distal convoluted tubule and collecting tubule. Each part is lined with a special cell and there are brush borders, cell inclusions and exotic staining reactions. In addition the kidney consumes a considerable amount of oxygen doing its job. By contrast, the structure of the lung unit is remarkably simple (figure 1) and the

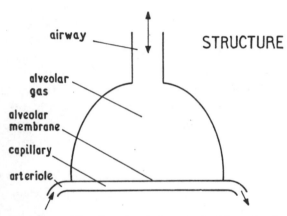

Figure 1. The functional lung unit. The alveolar membrane across which gas exchange occurs, has alveolar gas on one side and pulmonary capillary blood on the other. Gas is brought to the alveoli by the bronchi and blood to the capillaries by arterioles.

reasons for these differences in structure are the differences in function. The kidney is concerned with regulating the concentration of a variety of substances in the blood—many ions, urea and other solutes, and as part of this job it uses energy to pump sodium ions against concentration gradients. On the other hand, the lung as a gas exchanger is chiefly concerned with only two substances, oxygen and carbon dioxide, and these move by passive physical diffusion. This means that they move from a region of high partial pressure to a region of low partial pressure just as water runs down-hill. For this reason, the lung tissue does no work on these gases and it consumes little oxygen itself. Thus the structure of the lung unit is simple because its function is simple: it merely brings blood and air very close together so that gases can exchange by passive diffusion.

To all this, the pathologist may retort that the structure of the lung is not at all like figure 1 in that the large bronchi divide into smaller bronchioles which lead into terminal and respiratory bronchioles and finally into alveolar ducts from which the alveoli bud. This is true, but from a functional standpoint, the lung can be divided into two volumes: the conducting airways where no gas exchange with blood occurs, and the 'alveolar gas' volume where gas is continually exchanging with blood. The precise division in anatomical terms between these two functional compartments is not yet known but the 'alveolar gas' volume includes the alveoli themselves, the alveolar ducts and probably the respiratory bronchioles.

Now let us put some figures for the volumes and flows of gas and blood on this lung unit. If we assume that all the units are the same, figure 1 can be used to denote the whole organ as well as a single unit. Figure 2 shows that the total volume of the conducting airways is about 150 ml. (These and the following numbers are typical values only and there is considerable variation.) The total lung gas volume at the end of a normal expiration (functional residual capacity) is about 2,500 to 3,000 ml. Thus the conducting volume is a remarkably small proportion of the active gas exchanging volume but nevertheless as we shall see, a considerable proportion of inspired gas is wasted in the bronchi. By contrast with the large alveolar gas volume, the volume of blood undergoing gas exchange in the pulmonary capillaries is only about 70 ml.

Turning now to the movement of gas and blood, suppose the tidal volume is 500 ml and the number of breaths each minute is 15. The total volume of air passing the lips each minute (in one direction) is therefore $500 \times 15 = 7{,}500$ ml/min; this is called the minute volume. Of this 500 ml of inspired air, 150 ml remains in the airways (anatomic dead space) and takes no part in gas exchange; this volume can therefore be disregarded in the ensuing discussion. The remainder of the 500 ml, that is 350 ml, enters the

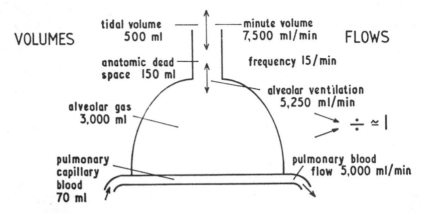

Figure 2. Lung unit with the volumes of gas and blood for the whole organ (both lungs). Numbers are typical values only and there is considerable variation. Note that the normal ratio of ventilation to blood flow is about 1.

alveolar volume. This is the volume which matters for gas exchange; the volume per minute $350 \times 15 = 5{,}250$ ml/min is called the alveolar ventilation. (Conventionally, the alveolar ventilation is strictly the volume of this gas when it leaves the alveoli which is usually slightly smaller because less carbon dioxide is given out than oxygen is taken in.) On the blood side of the alveolar membrane, the total pulmonary capillary flow is the same as the cardiac output, say 5,000 ml/min. Note the important fact that the total volume of fresh gas (alveolar ventilation) and the total volume of fresh blood brought to the alveolar membrane each minute are approximately the same. Thus the normal ventilation-perfusion ratio is about 1.

Perfect lung

A convenient way of approaching the normal transport of oxygen in the body and disturbances of this normal pattern by disease is to look at the gradual fall in oxygen partial pressure from air to tissues. In this way, we can compare the performance of the normal lung and the diseased lung with that of a perfect gas exchanger.

Figure 3 shows the oxygen partial pressures for a perfect lung. The total atmospheric pressure is about 760 mmHg and of this 20.9% is due to oxygen. Thus the P_{O_2} of air is 20.9% of 760 = 159 mmHg. (P_{O_2} means partial pressure of oxygen, P representing pressure). Actually as the air is inhaled, it becomes saturated with water vapour at body temperature so that from the total dry gas pressure we must subtract the partial pressure of water vapour (47 mmHg).

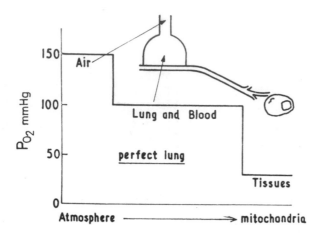

Figure 3. The perfect lung. Note that alveolar gas and arterial blood have the same oxygen tension. The large 'step' of some 50 mmHg between inspired and alveolar gas is determined by the balance between oxygen removal from alveolar gas by the blood and its replenishment by ventilation. (Modified from Payne, J. P. & Hill, D. W. (1966). *Oxygen measurements in blood and tissues and their significance.* J. & A. Churchill).

The P_{O_2} of moist inspired gas is therefore 20.9% of (760 − 47) = 149 mmHg (say 150 mmHg).

Figure 3 shows that in the perfect lung, the P_{O_2} in alveolar gas is much less than in inspired gas. This is because oxygen is continually being removed from this gas by the blood and carbon dioxide added. Indeed if it were not for the fact that alveolar ventilation continually replenishes the oxygen and removes carbon dioxide, the P_{O_2} would become lower and lower. As it is, a balance is struck between the rate at which oxygen is removed and the rate at which it is replenished giving an alveolar P_{O_2} of about

100 mmHg. If alveolar ventilation is reduced for the same oxygen consumption, the alveolar P_{O_2} falls, and similarly if the alveolar ventilation is increased (oxygen uptake constant), the alveolar P_{O_2} rises.

Note that even in this perfect oxygen transport system, one-third of the inspired P_{O_2} is lost before the oxygen reaches the arterial blood. It is worth pausing for a moment to compare the mammalian lung in this respect with the gill of the fish. It has been shown that the flows of inspired water and blood are in opposite directions in fish gills so that blood leaving a gill capillary is brought very close to fresh water entering the gill. The result is that, in principle, arterial blood can have the same P_{O_2} as the inspired water. Thus the large fall of P_{O_2} between inspired air and arterial blood which exists even in a perfect mammalian lung (figure 3) is avoided. A disadvantage of the arrangement in the fish is the vulnerability to brief exposure to a hypoxic environment because if the inspired P_{O_2} falls, the arterial P_{O_2} follows closely. By contrast, the alveolar gas volume in the mammalian lung is a useful store of oxygen which buffers the animal against short periods of breath-holding.

Figure 3 shows that the tissue P_{O_2} is much less than the arterial blood P_{O_2}. When the blood reaches the systemic capillaries, oxygen moves out into the cells and eventually to the mitochondria where it is used. Again movement is by simple physical diffusion from an area of high partial pressure to one of low partial pressure and there is evidence that the intracellular P_{O_2} may be very low, possibly less than 1 mmHg. In fact, the line marked 'tissues' in figure 3 is a great over-simplification because the P_{O_2} varies between different types of tissue and between adjacent parts of the same tissue. However it serves as a reminder that the arterial blood P_{O_2} is one link in the chain which eventually connects the air to the mitochondria.

Hypoventilation

Figure 4 introduces the first important cause of hypoxaemia, that is hypoventilation. We have seen that the alveolar P_{O_2} depends on a balance between the rate at which oxygen is removed from the lung by the blood and the rate at which it is replenished by alveolar ventilation. If ventilation is reduced, alveolar hypoxia and therefore arterial hypoxaemia must follow. It is clear that hypoxaemia due to hypoventilation may occur although the lung itself is normal. Causes include depression of the respiratory centre by drugs or anaesthesia, damage to the medulla by disease,

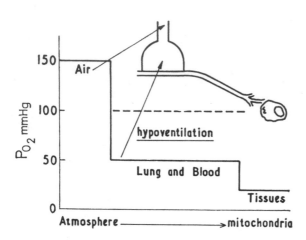

Figure 4. Hypoventilation. The difference between the oxygen tensions of inspired and alveolar gas is abnormally large because the rate of replenishment of the oxygen in alveolar gas has been reduced, while the rate at which it is removed by the blood remains unchanged.

diseases affecting the nerve supply to the muscles of the thorax or the muscles themselves, injury to the chest wall and obstruction to the upper airways. An important feature of hypoventilation as a cause of hypoxia is that because the lung itself is often normal, the prognosis is excellent if the precipitating cause can be removed. The defective gas exchange which occurs in hypoventilation is dealt with in more detail on p. 104 (figure 51).

In practice, the normal lung falls short of the perfect lung shown in figure 3 in three respects each of which may become a cause of hypoxaemia in disease. These are diffusion, shunt and

B

ventilation-perfusion ratio inequality. These defects show as discrete falls in the P_{O_2} so that the net result is that a lower P_{O_2} is available to the tissues. In the normal lung, these defects are small and their contributions to arterial hypoxaemia barely measurable, but in the diseased lung they may result in profound hypoxaemia.

Diffusion

Oxygen moves across the gas-blood interface by passive diffusion because the partial pressure in the alveolar gas is higher than that in the blood. Figure 5A shows the way in which the P_{O_2} rises in the blood as it flows along a pulmonary capillary when the lung is breathing air. The P_{O_2} of alveolar gas is about 100 mmHg; the P_{O_2} of mixed venous blood (blood in the pulmonary artery) is about 40 mmHg. When a corpuscle enters the capillary, it 'sees' a P_{O_2} of 100 mmHg on the other side of the alveolar membrane less than 1 micron away. Thus there is a driving pressure of $(100 - 40) = 60$ mmHg between gas and blood with the result that oxygen moves rapidly across the thin interface, and the P_{O_2} in the blood rises quickly. This rise in blood P_{O_2} now reduces the driving pressure so the rate at which oxygen moves across the membrane becomes less. The result is that the blood P_{O_2} rises in a curve.

The precise shape of this curve is difficult to determine but is unimportant in the present context. Thus the shape of the oxygen dissociation curve (figure 27A) has a large effect. It is also known that the rate at which oxygen moves across the alveolar membrane depends not only on the diffusion properties of the interface itself but also on the rate of chemical combination of oxygen with haemoglobin which itself varies with the P_{O_2} of the blood. In addition, the larger the volume of blood in the pulmonary capillaries, the faster the oxygen can move across.

Such complicating factors do not affect the present argument and two features of figure 5A should be emphasised. One is that the P_{O_2} of the blood becomes very nearly equal to that of the gas by the time the end of the capillary is reached. Theoretically a

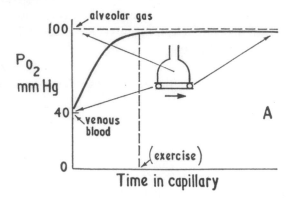

Figure 5A. Diagram of the way in which the P_{O_2} rises as the blood flows along the pulmonary capillary. Blood enters the capillary with a P_{O_2} of 40 mmHg and this rises rapidly until it is very close to the P_{O_2} of alveolar gas, 100 mmHg (typical values only). Note that when the lung breathes air, equilibration between gas and blood is nearly complete after one third of the time available, and that the P_{O_2} difference between alveolar gas and blood at the end of the capillary is exceedingly small. During exercise, the available time may be reduced to a third (dashed line) but equilibration is still almost complete. The alveolar P_{O_2} may rise on exercise.

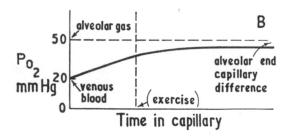

Figure 5B. Changes in capillary P_{O_2} when the lung breathes a low oxygen mixture which reduces the alveolar gas P_{O_2} to 50 mmHg. Now the rate of rise of blood P_{O_2} is much slower and there is an appreciable P_{O_2} difference between gas and blood at the end of the capillary. This difference is exaggerated on exercise because the time available for equilibration is reduced.

small difference must remain but in practice this is immeasurably small in the normal lung. Nevertheless, this alveolar end-capillary difference is shown as a small 'step' in the P_{O_2} line in figure 6. Secondly the P_{O_2} of the blood has nearly reached that of the gas after only one-third of the available time in the capillary. Thus in the normal resting lung, there are great reserves of diffusion. These reserves are highlighted during exercise which stresses the diffusion

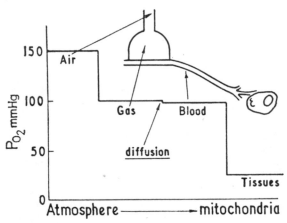

Figure 6. The perfect lung modified to show the effect of the diffusion barrier across the alveolar membrane. The P_{O_2} of blood in the capillary never quite reaches the P_{O_2} of alveolar gas thus introducing a 'step'. In the normal lung when breathing air, this step is immeasurably small but in disease it may become significant.

ability of the lung. The effect of exercise is to reduce the time spent by the blood in the pulmonary capillary and it is clear that even if the time available for diffusion is reduced to one-third of normal, the normal lung is able to oxygenate the blood effectively. The rise of alveolar P_{O_2} which tends to occur on exercise also helps the diffusion process.

A more exacting test of the diffusion ability of the lung is alveolar hypoxia. Figure 5B shows how the P_{O_2} of the capillary blood rises under these conditions. Suppose the alveolar P_{O_2} is only 50 mmHg because the lung is breathing a low oxygen mixture and the P_{O_2} of the mixed venous blood is 20 mmHg. Now a corpuscle entering the capillary is exposed to a driving pressure of only 30 mmHg (as opposed to 60 mmHg in figure 5A) and the rate of movement of oxygen across the alveolar membrane is correspondingly slower. Thus as figure 5B shows, an appreciable difference between the P_{O_2} of gas and blood may remain at the end of the capillary. Furthermore if alveolar hypoxia is combined with heavy exercise, the reduction of the time available for diffusion under these difficult conditions exaggerates the diffusion defect. This mechanism is responsible for some of the severe hypoxaemia in acclimatized normal subjects during heavy exercise at very high altitudes.

The diffusion process under normal conditions (figure 5A) is enhanced by the shape of the oxygen dissociation curve (figure 27A). Because the curve is so flat when the P_{O_2} is high, most of the oxygen has passed across the interface before the capillary blood P_{O_2} has approached close to the alveolar P_{O_2}. Thus the large driving gradient is maintained until almost all the oxygen is transferred. By contrast, the lung is operating on the steeper straighter portion of the dissociation curve during alveolar hypoxia (figure 5B) and this advantage is not obtained.

Lung disease may further impede the diffusion of oxygen across the alveolar membrane. There are conditions such as diffuse interstitial fibrosis, sarcoidosis, asbestosis, and alveolar carcinomatosis where microscopically, the alveolar blood-gas barrier appears to be thickened, and it is possible that some of the arterial hypoxaemia in these conditions is caused by defective diffusion. As shown above, difficulties with diffusion are particularly prone to occur when the oxygen uptake is increased or the alveolar P_{O_2} is low so that typically these patients often become dramatically cyanosed on exercise or when given a low oxygen mixture to breathe. Thus a woman in her thirties may be seen at out-patients to be somewhat breathless at rest with shallow rapid breathing, and perhaps she is slightly cyanosed. When she walks up a flight of stairs, she becomes very breathless and very much bluer; her arterial P_{CO_2} tends to be low. Such a patient may have impaired diffusion.

The term 'alveolar-capillary block' was coined for this condition and the phrase nicely fits the histological picture and trips lightly off the tongue. However the term should be used with discretion for several reasons. One is that most of the arterial hypoxaemia in these patients is now known to be due to ventilation-perfusion ratio inequality rather than to impaired diffusion (see later in this chapter and in chapter 3). Calculations have suggested that the observed degree of thickening of the blood-gas barrier is insufficient to interfere seriously with oxygen diffusion without causing considerable inequality of ventilation and blood flow [8], and this has been shown to be present in these conditions [6, 8, 22]. Again the term focusses all the attention on the alveolar membrane although much of the diffusion resistance depends on reaction rates in the red cell.

Thus in summary, impaired diffusion due to pulmonary disease such as diffuse interstitial fibrosis probably does occur and when it does, its effects are much accentuated by exercise or the inhalation of a low oxygen mixture. However, ventilation-perfusion ratio inequality is a more important cause of the arterial hypoxaemia even in diseases where the alveolar membrane is thickened. Ways of distinguishing between these two mechanisms are discussed in chapter 6.

Shunt

The second respect in which the actual lung falls short of the perfect lung shown in figure 3 is that there are contributions to the arterial blood which have not been through ventilated areas of lung. In the normal subject, these include part of the bronchial venous blood which finds its way into the pulmonary veins and thence into the systemic circulation, Thebesian veins which drain from the myocardium direct into the left side of the heart, and possibly a few small direct connections between the pulmonary arteries and veins. The addition of this poorly oxygenated blood to the pulmonary venous blood results in a second 'step' in the P_{O_2} line as shown in figure 7. In the normal subject, these contributions are equivalent to only 1–2% of the cardiac output bypassing the lung, and the resulting fall in arterial P_{O_2} is only some 5 mmHg which is hardly measurable. Thus under normal conditions, the effect of this shunt on the arterial P_{O_2} is negligible.

In disease however, right to left shunts may result in severe hypoxaemia. The commonest group of patients in the wards today to which this applies are the patients with congenital heart disease such as the tetralogy of Fallot. Patients with atrial and ventricular septal defects who develop pulmonary hypertension may also

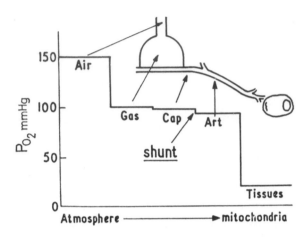

Figure 7. The perfect lung modified to show the depression of blood P_{O_2} by the diffusion and shunt effects. The latter arises because of additions to the arterial blood of blood which has not been through ventilated areas of lung. (Modified from Payne, J. P. & Hill, D. W. (1966). *Oxygen measurements in blood and tissues and their significance.* J. & A. Churchill.)

develop large right to left shunts. Pulmonary conditions such as atelectasis, pulmonary oedema and abnormal arterio-venous connections through fistulae may also result in arterial hypoxaemia from this cause.

Ventilation-perfusion ratio inequality

So far we have considered three of the four causes of hypoxaemia— hypoventilation, impaired diffusion, and shunts. The first can be looked upon as an exaggeration of the normal difference of 50 mmHg or so between inspired and alveolar gas which exists in the normal lung (figures 3 and 4). The second two may be looked upon as imperfections of the perfect lung though they cause negligible interference with gas exchange under normal conditions (figures 6 and 7).

The last cause we must consider is by far the most important but also the most difficult to understand. It is the mechanism which is responsible for most of the hypoxaemia in the general medical wards, for example, the hypoxaemia of chronic obstructive lung disease, pneumonia and pulmonary fibrosis. In this section, the notion will be introduced to be taken up in more detail in chapter 4.

We have assumed until now that all the lung units behave in an identical way. Thus the perfect lung of figures 2 and 3 is simply a magnified version of the simple lung unit of figure 1. In practice, this is not so because the share of the total blood flow going to each unit is different as also is its share of the total ventilation. The reasons for these differences are discussed in chapter 2. Briefly, on the one hand, the weight of the column of blood in the upright lung increases the perfusing pressure and therefore the blood flow at the base, and on the other hand, the weight of the lung itself affects the pleural pressure down the lung and thus the regional ventilation. The upshot is that the blood flow increases rapidly down the lung; the ventilation also increases but much more slowly. Thus at the apex of the upright lung, there are alveoli which have almost no blood flow and a moderate ventilation, while at the base the blood flow is much larger but the ventilation is only slightly increased. The result is that the ventilation-perfusion ratio decreases down the lung.

We shall see in chapter 3 that the ventilation-perfusion ratio is the key variable controlling gas exchange so that because it changes down the lung, there are inevitable regional differences in alveolar gas P_{O_2} (figure 26). Thus the P_{O_2} is more than 130 mmHg near the apex but less than 90 mmHg near the base, and the P_{O_2} of capillary blood draining from these areas will be similar (in fact, very slightly lower because of the diffusion 'step'). For this reason, we cannot represent the P_{O_2} of alveolar gas and end-capillary blood by single lines as in figure 7, but must put in a range of values as in figure 8. Note that the block of lines representing the P_{O_2} of end-capillary blood is displaced slightly downwards to draw attention to the small diffusion gradient in each alveolus.

While the range of alveolar P_{O_2} in the upright lung is of some interest, the effect of this ventilation-perfusion ratio inequality on the P_{O_2} of mixed capillary blood is of much greater importance.

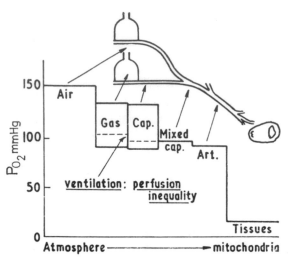

Figure 8. The perfect lung modified to show the effects of ventilation-perfusion ratio ($\dot{V}A/\dot{Q}$) inequality, diffusion and shunt. Because blood flow and ventilation are unevenly distributed from the apex to the base of the upright lung, there is a range of P_{O_2} in alveolar gas (and capillary blood). In addition, the P_{O_2} of mixed capillary blood is depressed because it is weighed by contributions from the base of the lung which have a low P_{O_2}. The diffusion and shunt effects result in further lowering of the arterial P_{O_2}. (Modified from Payne, J. P. & Hill, D. W. (1966). *Oxygen measurements in blood and tissues and their significance.* J. & A. Churchill.)

It transpires that even if the overall blood flow and ventilation of the lung remain the same when the unevenness occurs, the result of the unevenness is to depress the P_{O_2} of the blood draining from it. Basically this is because the pulmonary venous blood is weighted by contributions from the lower part of the lung where the blood flow is high and the P_{O_2} is low. Thus the mere fact that the blood flow and ventilation do not meet in the correct proportions has the effect of lowering the blood P_{O_2} just as hypoventilation, diffusion, and the shunt effects do. This is the main theme of this monograph and is taken up in detail in chapter 4.

In the normal lung, the depression of the blood P_{O_2} by ventilation-perfusion ratio inequality amounts to less than 5 mm of Hg and is therefore hardly measurable. It is of the same order as that caused by the shunt effect (figure 7). However, in disease the mechanism is often of great importance, cutting the arterial P_{O_2} to perhaps half of its normal value of about 100 mmHg. In addition, the ventilation-perfusion ratio inequality also interferes with carbon dioxide transfer so that carbon dioxide retention may follow. This mechanism is responsible for the arterial hypoxaemia of the great bulk of lung disease and it is the commonest cause of cyanosis in the general medical wards.

Chapter 2

Inequality of blood flow and ventilation in the normal lung

This chapter deals with the causes and some consequences of the uneven distribution of blood flow and ventilation in the normal lung. It is something of a diversion from the main topic of gas exchange so that some readers may choose to accept the normal pattern of ventilation-perfusion ratio inequality shown in figure 21 and move directly to chapter 3.

Distribution of blood flow

The subject of the topographical distribution of blood flow in the lung is both old and new; old because as long ago as 1887, Johannes Orth considered that the weight of the column of blood in the erect lungs might cause apical anaemia, and new because it was only with the introduction of radioactive gases that it became possible to make quantitative measurements of regional blood flow. One such technique is shown in figure 9A.

The subject is seated and pairs of scintillation counters examine antero-posterior cores of lung. When the subject inhales a single breath of carbon dioxide labelled with radioactive oxygen, the rise in counting rate is determined by the ventilation of the lung in the counting field and its volume. During a subsequent 15 second breath-holding period, radioactive gas can only be removed by the pulmonary blood flow. Thus the slope of the counting rate tracing (clearance rate) is a measure of regional blood flow.

This procedure while simple for the subject requires a cyclotron in the vicinity to supply the radioactive oxygen because its half

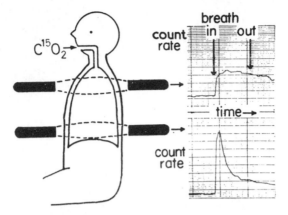

Figure 9A. Method of measuring regional ventilation and blood flow in the lung with radioactive carbon dioxide. The subject takes a single breath of labelled gas and holds his breath for some 15 seconds. The counting rate at the end of inspiration is proportional to the ventilation of the lung in the counting field and its volume, while the slope of the tracing during breath-holding (clearance rate) measures the regional blood flow. (From the *British Medical Bulletin.*)

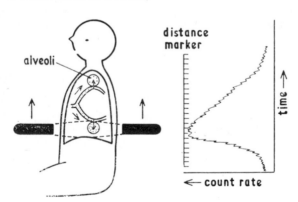

Figure 9B. Method of measuring regional blood flow with radioactive xenon. A saline solution of the gas is injected into an arm vein and when it reaches the lung, the xenon is evolved into alveolar gas because of its low solubility. During breath-holding, both lungs are scanned from bottom to top with pairs of counters.

life is only 2 minutes. A method more generally available because it uses the reactor-produced xenon—133 (half life 5 days) is shown in figure 9B. A saline solution of radioactive xenon is injected into the superior vena cava through a polythene catheter and as the labelled blood passes through the lung, the xenon is evolved into alveolar gas because of its low solubility. It remains there during the breath-holding period and advantage is taken of this stable situation to measure the distribution of intrapulmonary radio-activity with a gamma camera or with moving counters. A second measurement is made after distributing the radioactive xenon uniformly throughout the alveolar gas by rebreathing and a comparison of the two scans gives the blood flow per unit of alveolar volume. Ventilation may be measured with a single breath of the gas just as in the radioactive carbon dioxide method; alternatively the rate of wash-in of xenon can be recording during normal breathing with the subject connected to a spirometer.

Figure 10 shows the distribution of blood flow in the normal upright human lung as found from many pooled measurements in 16 normal volunteers using radioactive carbon dioxide. It can be

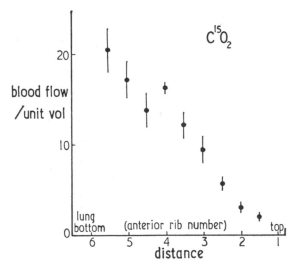

Figure 10. Distribution of blood flow in the normal upright lung as measured with radioactive carbon dioxide. Data from 16 normal subjects; means and standard errors of clearance rates. Note that blood flow decreases steadily from the bottom to the top of the lung there being virtually no flow at the apex. (From the *Journal of Applied Physiology*.)

seen that there is a steady fall in blood flow per unit volume with rib number and therefore distance, from the bottom to the top of the lung and that flow is virtually nil at the apex. Essentially the same pattern of distribution is found with radioactive xenon.

This normal distribution of pulmonary blood flow is affected by changes of posture and by exercise. When the subject lies supine, the apical zone blood flow increases but the basal zone flow remains virtually unchanged with the result that the distribution from apex to base becomes almost uniform. In this posture, blood flow in the posterior regions of the lung exceeds flow in the anterior parts. Measurements on men suspended upside-down show that apical blood flow may much exceed basal flow in this position. On mild exercise, both upper and lower zone blood flow increase but the upper increases more than the lower, so that the flow becomes more even.

Circulatory changes occurring with heart disease also affect the distribution of blood flow. Thus in diseases which increase pulmonary blood flow such as left-to-right intracardiac shunts, flow is more evenly distributed than in the normal lung and the resulting pattern is similar to that found during exercise. In conditions in which the pulmonary arterial pressure is increased because of increased vascular resistance but pulmonary blood flow is not necessarily raised, flow is again more evenly distributed. In diseases which raise the pulmonary venous pressure, for example mitral stenosis, the distribution of blood flow becomes more uniform with moderate disease, but later in the presence of severe pulmonary venous hypertention, the normal distribution may be inverted so that more flow goes to the upper than the lower zones.

Cause of the distribution of blood flow

An analysis of the role of the various intrathoracic pressures in determining the distribution of blood flow in man is hardly feasible because of the difficulty of changing one pressure at a time and measuring the flow distribution under rigorously controlled conditions. For this reason, the problem has been studied in an isolated lung preparation where these conditions could be met. The left lung of a dog was removed and mounted upright in a Perspex box after cannulating the pulmonary artery, veins and bronchus. The lung was ventilated with negative pressure and perfused by a non-pulsatile flow of warm venous blood from a second dog. Many features of this lung such as its ability to exchange gas, its pulmonary vascular resistance, its elastic properties and its increase in vasomotor tone when hypoxic, showed that its function was normal in many respects for some hours at least.

Figure 11 shows an example of the distribution of blood flow found in this preparation using the radioactive xenon technique.

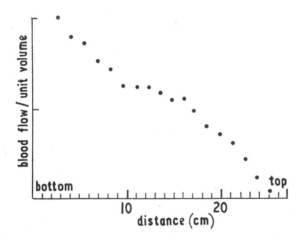

Figure 11. Distribution of blood flow in an isolated lung with a normal pulmonary arterial pressure and low venous pressure. Note the similarity to the distribution in the human lung shown in figure 10. (From the *Journal of Applied Physiology*.)

It can be seen that there was an approximately linear decrease in blood flow with distance up the lung and that flow fell almost to zero near the apex. The similarity to the normal distribution of blood flow in the upright human lung shown in figure 10 is apparent. For the measurement shown in figure 11, the pulmonary arterial pressure was 32 cm H_2O referred to the bottom of the lung which measured 27 cm in vertical height, and the alveolar pressure was atmospheric.

How do changes in the pulmonary arterial, venous and alveolar pressures affect this distribution of blood flow? Figure 12 shows the flow distribution under precisely the same conditions as those of figure 11 except that the pulmonary arterial pressure was

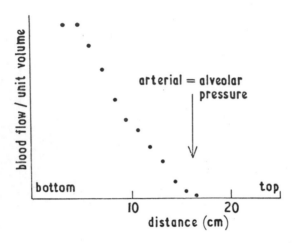

Figure 12. Effect of reducing the pulmonary arterial pressure on the distribution of blood flow shown in figure 11. Blood flow still decreases steadily from the bottom of the lung but falls to zero some two thirds of the way up the lung. The unperfused zone is above the level where arterial pressure equals alveolar pressure. (From the *Journal of Applied Physiology*.)

reduced to 16 cm H_2O (referred to the bottom of the lung) by lowering the blood flow from about 500 to 200 ml/min. It can be seen that blood flow again decreased approximately linearly with distance up the lung but this time it fell to zero some two-thirds of the way up the lung. By allowing for the decrease in pulmonary arterial pressure of 1 cm H_2O/cm distance up the lung (hydrostatic effect), the level at which arterial pressure equalled alveolar pressure could be calculated and this is shown in figure 12. Note that this calculation neglects the pressure drop along the arteries caused by flow but that this error becomes progressively smaller as the no-flow level is approached. Figure 12 shows a close agreement between the no-flow level and that at which arterial pressure equalled alveolar pressure and this was confirmed in a series of measurements in which both arterial and alveolar pressure were varied. Thus the result of increasing arterial pressure was always to raise the no-flow level while the effect of increasing alveolar pressure was always to depress it.

For figures 11 and 12, the pulmonary venous pressure was held low and figure 13 is an example in another lung of the effect

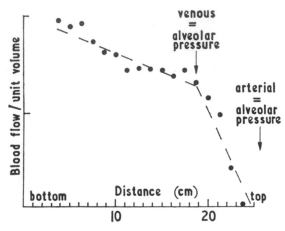

Figure 13. Effect of increasing the pulmonary venous pressure on the distribution of blood flow in the isolated lung. Blood flow has become more uniform in the part of the lung below the level at which venous pressure equalled alveolar pressure. (From the *Journal of Applied Physiology.*)

of raising the venous pressure. It can be seen that the result was to make the distribution of flow in the lower part of the lung more even although in some preparations, this was much less marked. In the diagram, a dashed line has been drawn with an inflexion at the level where venous pressure equalled alveolar pressure because other measurements show that the venous pressure only affects the distribution of flow below this level.

It is possible to draw a simple model which accounts for these observed distributions of blood flow (figure 14) and it is interesting

c

to keep this in the mind's eye when looking at a chest radiograph. The lung is divided into 3 zones by the relative magnitudes of the pulmonary arterial, venous and alveolar pressures.

In *zone 1*, arterial pressure is less than alveolar pressure and there is no flow. Presumably this is because thin-walled collapsible vessels (for example, the capillaries) are directly exposed to alveolar pressure. Observations on rapidly frozen lung sections

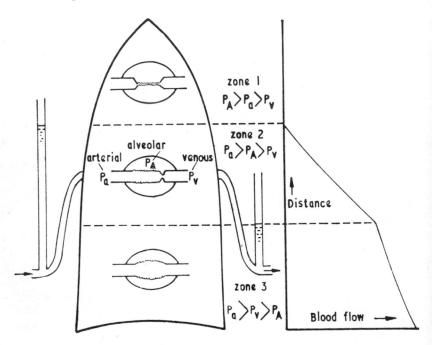

Figure 14. Scheme which accounts for the distribution of blood flow in the isolated lung. In *zone 1*, alveolar pressure exceeds arterial pressure and no flow occurs presumably because collapsible vessels are directly exposed to alveolar pressure. In *zone 2*, arterial pressure exceeds alveolar pressure, but alveolar exceeds venous pressure. Here the vessels behave like Starling resistors (figure 15) and flow is determined by the arterial-alveolar pressure difference which steadily increases down the zone. In *zone 3*, venous pressure now exceeds alveolar pressure and flow is determined by the arterial-venous pressure difference which is constant down the lung. However the pressure across the walls of the vessels increases down the zone, so that their calibre increases and so does flow. (From the *Journal of Applied Physiology*.)

from this zone confirm that the capillaries are collapsed and virtually bloodless [10]. Note particularly that in man, the pulmonary artery pressure is sufficient to raise blood to the apex of the lung so that no *zone 1* is present under normal conditions (figure 10).

In *zone 2*, arterial pressure exceeds alveolar pressure, but alveolar exceeds venous pressure. Here each vessel apparently behaves like the resistor in a Starling heart-lung preparation, that is a collapsible tube surrounded by a pressure chamber

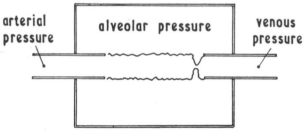

Figure 15. Starling resistor which consists of a collapsible tube in a pressure chamber. The behaviour of this model is thought to explain the increase in blood flow down *zone 2* of the lung (figure 14).

(figure 15). This device has the interesting property that when the chamber (alveolar) pressure exceeds the downstream (venous) pressure, flow is determined not by the upstream-downstream pressure difference but by the upstream-chamber pressure difference. The reason for this is that the thin tube offers no resistance to the collapsing pressure so that the pressure inside the tube is the same as the pressure outside. The result is that the pressure gradient responsible for flow is the perfusing pressure minus chamber pressure. The collapsible tube actually develops a constriction in its downstream end (where the pressure inside the tube is least). In the lung, alveolar pressure is the same at every level while arterial pressure steadily increases down the lung because of the hydrostatic effect. Thus the increase of flow with distance down *zone 2* is satisfactorily explained.

In *zone 3*, venous pressure now exceeds alveolar pressure, the collapsible tube is held open and flow is determined by the arterial-venous pressure difference in the ordinary way. Again an increase in flow with distance down the lung is observed (figure 14) and at first sight the reason for this is not clear since the arterial-venous pressure difference is constant down the lung. However while the pressure inside the small vessels increases down the zone (hydrostatic effect) the pressure outside is constant since it is alveolar pressure. Thus the transmural pressure increases down the zone and if we assume that parts of the vessels are not only collapsible but distensible, then their flow resistance will decrease down the zone. Measurements on capillaries in rapidly frozen lung sections from this region show that capillary width does increase with distance down *zone 3* [10].

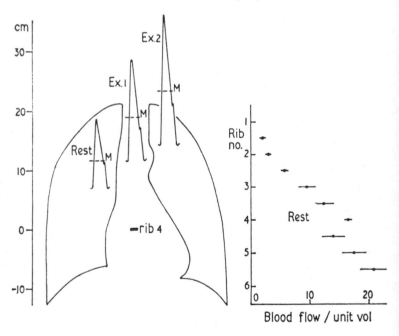

Figure 16. Pulmonary arterial pressures in the upright human lung at rest and two levels of exercise. Data of Bevegard *et al.* [1]. If blood rises only to the level at which arterial pressure equals alveolar pressure, this diagram suggests that the extreme apex of the lung may be unperfused at rest but on exercise blood flow will become more uniform. M is the mean pressure. The right hand graph shows the observed distribution of blood flow at rest (same data as in figure 10); agreement with that predicted from the pulmonary arterial pressure is good.

In the human lung, the pressure in the pulmonary artery is very pulsatile, but probably only about one-third of the pulse wave is transmitted to the small collapsible vessels [15, 16]. Figure 16 shows measurements of pulmonary artery pressure in seated normal volunteers at rest and two levels of exercise (oxygen consumptions of one and two litres/min respectively) [1]. It suggests that the extreme apex of the lung is unperfused at rest though probably in most people pulmonary arterial pressure is just sufficient to raise blood to the top of the lung. On exercise, appreciable increases in pulmonary arterial pressure occur so that the differences in blood flow down the lung then become much less marked.

The relations between pulmonary arterial, alveolar and venous pressures and the consequent behaviour of the capillaries apparently explain many of the distributions of blood flow observed in man. However recently it has been found that the distribution is considerably altered at low lung volumes [11]. Figure 17 shows that while at total lung capacity, blood flow increases down most of the lung, at functional residual capacity, there is an area of reduced blood flow near the base, while at residual volume, blood flow is actually higher at the second rib level than at the base.

These changes can be explained by the contribution to vascular resistance made by the larger blood vessels at low lung volumes. Figure 18 shows that we can distinguish between 'alveolar' vessels, including capillaries which are exposed to alveolar pressure, and 'extra-alveolar vessels' which are surrounded by a negative pressure which depends on the state of the lung inflation [20]. At high lung volumes, these larger vessels are pulled open and their vascular resistance is low; at low lung volumes, they contribute a high resistance. At the base of the lung at functional residual capacity, the lung parenchyma is believed to be poorly expanded (figure 20) so that the resistance of the extra-alveolar vessels is high and blood flow is therefore reduced. This reduction is not seen at total lung capacity because then all the lung is well expanded. At residual volume, the resistance of the extra-alveolar vessels dominates and the distribution of blood flow is unaffected by the hydrostatic gradient within the vessels.

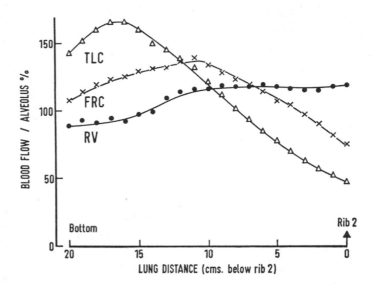

Figure 17. Effect of lung volume on the distribution of blood flow in man. Note that while at total lung capacity (TLC) blood flow increases down most of the lung, there is a region of reduced blood flow near the base at functional residual capacity (FRC), and this spreads up the lung at residual volume (RV). (From *Respiration Physiology*.)

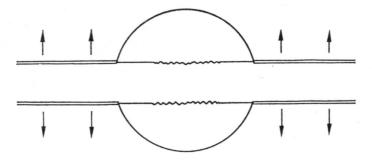

Figure 18. Diagram to emphasize the difference between 'alveolar' vessels (including capillaries) exposed to alveolar pressure and the larger 'extra-alveolar' vessels (perhaps over 100 microns in diameter) which are surrounded by a negative pressure generated by the expansion of the lung parenchyma. When lung volume is low, the resistance of these vessels is high. (From *Respiration Physiology*.)

Distribution of ventilation

While blood flow per unit volume decreases rapidly up the normal lung (figure 10) the change in ventilation is not nearly so marked. Figure 19 shows the normal distribution of ventilation in the upright human lung as found using radioactive xenon [3]. It can be seen that ventilation per unit of alveolar volume decreases with distance up the lung, just as blood flow does, but that the rate of change of ventilation is much less (about one-third that of blood flow).

Change of posture affects the distribution of ventilation as it does blood flow. When normal subjects lie supine, the difference in ventilation between the anatomical upper and lower zones is abolished [3]. Furthermore, it has been shown that in the inverted lung, the apex ventilates better than the base, so that the normal pattern is reversed.

Interesting observations have been made on the relative rates of expansion of the upper and lower zones of the upright lung when the subject breathes in (in steps) from residual volume, that is

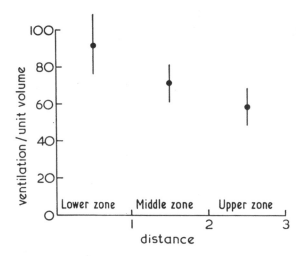

Figure 19. Distribution of ventilation in the upright human lung. Data of Bryan *et al.* [3]. Means and standard errors. Note that ventilation decreases up the lung but that the rate of change is much less than for blood flow (compare figure 10). (From the *Journal of Applied Physiology.*)

after expelling as much air from the lungs as he can [17]. For these measurements, sufficient time was allowed at the end of each increase of volume to ensure that the lung had stopped moving. It was shown that when small amounts of gas were inspired from the residual volume position, the lower zones did not ventilate at all, so that all the gas went to the upper zones. However as the lung became expanded, the lower zones began to fill also, and by the time the lung volume had increased to about 20 % of its vital capacity, both upper and lower zones were inspiring at about the same rate. Thereafter, the lower zones filled more rapidly than the upper for the remainder of the full inspiration. This last pattern also applies to the normal tidal volumes of resting breathing when the lower zones ventilate more than the upper (figure 19).

Cause of the distribution of ventilation

It now appears that the uneven distribution of ventilation, like blood flow, is caused by gravity. Because the weight of the lung is supported partly by the chest wall and diaphragm, the intrapleural pressure is less negative at the bottom than the top. This has been confirmed by direct measurements in animals. As a consequence of these regional differences in expanding pressure, the distribution of ventilation is affected.

Figure 20A shows the differences in intrapleural and transpulmonary pressures which may exist down an upright lung which is 30 cm high at the end of a normal expiration. It can be seen that if the intrapleural pressure changes by 0.25 cm H_2O/cm of distance down the lung (a reasonable value from reported measurements), the total change in transpulmonary pressure from the top to bottom is 7.5 cm H_2O. This means that the upper and lower parts of the lung are operating on different portions of the pressure-volume curve so that the alveoli near the base are compressed and their volume is always smaller. In addition, the pressure-volume curve is not linear so that the base of the lung expands more than the apex. Both these effects will result in a larger ventilation per unit alveolar volume at the bottom of the upright lung compared with the top.

Figure 20B shows the pressures at residual volume, that is when as much gas as possible has been exhaled from the lung. Now the intrapleural pressure at the base actually exceeds the airway pressure and the alveoli are not ventilated because of airway collapse. Under these conditions, the apex of the lung ventilates better than the base. Thus this simple model explains the pattern of ventilation observed as the subject inhales in steps from residual volume [17] as described at the end of the last section. At abnormally low transpulmonary pressures (very small lung volumes), the base of the lung does not ventilate and all the inspired gas goes to the upper zones, whereas in the normal working range of pressures, the base ventilates more (per unit of

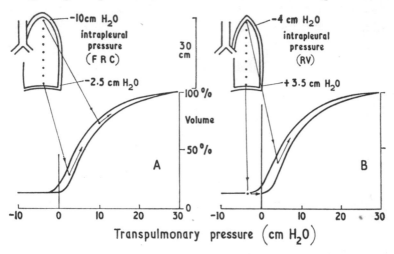

Figure 20. Effect of a gradient of intrapleural pressure up the lung on the distribution of ventilation. The pressure is assumed to fall at the rate of 0.25 cm H_2O/cm vertical distance. In A, at the beginning of a normal inspiration (FRC), the transpulmonary pressures at the apex and base are assumed to be 10 and 2.5 cm H_2O respectively. The two regions are therefore on different parts of the pressure-volume curve and the lung units at the base have a smaller initial volume and a larger change in volume than those at the apex [9]. Ventilation therefore decreases with distance up the lung (compare figure 19). By contrast, in B at residual volume (RV), the intrapleural pressure at the base may actually exceed airway pressure so that this region is not ventilated and the lung here is at its minimal volume.

pressure change) than the apex, and this pattern of inequality holds right up to maximal lung volumes.

Note that at residual volume, the alveoli at the base of the lung still contain some gas in spite of the fact that intrapleural exceeds alveolar pressure. This is because small airways just proximal to the alveoli close first trapping gas. For airway closure to occur in normal young subjects they must exhale well below functional residual volume, but many normal men over 60 years of age have some basal airways closed at the end of a normal expiration. The reason for this is that the elastic recoil of the lung diminishes with age and intrapleural pressure becomes less negative at a given lung volume. For the same reason, basal airway closure at functional residual capacity is common in pulmonary emphysema.

Distribution of ventilation-perfusion ratio

We have seen that both blood flow and ventilation change approximate linearly with distance up the normal upright lung (figures 10 and 19), and in figure 21 both distributions have been redrawn as simple linear relationships with distance. The curves have been smoothed out because from now on we shall be dealing with general patterns of distribution rather than exact figures. If we assume reasonable values such as 6 litres per minute for total blood flow and 5.1 litres per minute for total ventilation we can put in figures for blood flow and ventilation expressed as litres per minute per cent alveolar volume. Since both blood flow and ventilation are now in the same units, we can divide one by the other to get the ventilation-perfusion ratio.

Figure 21 shows that the ventilation-perfusion ratio is abnormally low (about 0.6) at the base of the lung, the overall value for the whole lung being 0.85. However it rises at first slowly and then rapidly as we go up the lung reaching high values (over 3.0) at the apex. In words, this means that the alveoli at the base of the lung are slightly over-perfused in relation to their ventilation whereas the alveoli at the apex are greatly under-perfused in relation to their ventilation. The degree of over-perfusion or

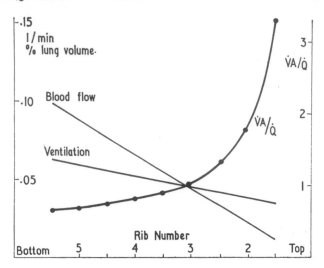

Figure 21. Distribution of ventilation, blood flow and ventilation-perfusion ratio up the normal upright lung. Straight lines have been drawn through the ventilation and blood flow data (figures 10 and 17). Because blood flow falls more rapidly then ventilation with distance up the lung, ventilation-perfusion ratio rises, slowly at first, then rapidly. This is the ventilation-perfusion ratio pattern which is used for many of the diagrams in chapters 3 and 4, the closed circles showing the ventilation-perfusion ratios of the 9 lung slices (see later).

under-ventilation is most conveniently expressed in terms of the ratio of ventilation to perfusion ($\dot{V}A/\dot{Q}$). It is this ratio which determines the gas exchange in any lung unit or region of the lung.

We shall use this pattern of ventilation-perfusion ratio inequality extensively in chapters 3 and 4 to examine its effect on regional gas exchange and overall gas exchange for the whole lung. The advantage of this approach is that because the ventilation-perfusion ratio changes in a regular manner up the lung, its influence on gas exchange can be mapped out and thus more easily grasped. This serves as an introduction to the more difficult notions of gas exchange in the diseased lung where ventilation-perfusion ratio inequality has more serious consequences but where the problems are much less amenable to a systematic approach.

Chapter 3

Ventilation-perfusion ratio inequality and regional gas exchange

Ventilation-perfusion ratio of the lung unit

In chapter 1, the function of the lung unit (figures 1 and 2) was discussed and it was shown that for gas exchange to occur, fresh inspired gas is brought to one side of the alveolar membrane by the alveolar ventilation, and blood is presented to the other side in the pulmonary capillary. It was also seen that under normal conditions, the P_{O_2} in the blood becomes very nearly equal to that of alveolar gas by the time the blood has reached the end of the capillary (figure 5A). The same is true for carbon dioxide and nitrogen, and from here on we shall assume complete equilibration between gas and blood in any alveolus.

We also saw that whereas the inspired P_{O_2} is about 150 mmHg, the P_{O_2} of alveolar gas and end-capillary blood is normally only about 100 mmHg, and this level is set by a balance between the rate at which fresh oxygen is brought in by the alveolar ventilation and the rate at which oxygen is removed by the blood. If the alveolar ventilation is increased and the rate of oxygen removal remains constant, the P_{O_2} of alveolar gas (and end-capillary blood) will rise. Conversely if the alveolar ventilation falls (oxygen uptake constant), the alveolar P_{O_2} also falls. In the same way, if the alveolar ventilation is held constant and the rate of oxygen removal is increased by raising the blood flow, the alveolar P_{O_2} will fall, and vice versa.

The way in which the P_{O_2} depends on the ventilation and blood flow is clarified by a simple model (figure 22). Suppose powdered dye is poured from a beaker into a mixing chamber through which water flows continuously. How does the concentration of dye

(P_{O_2}) in the chamber depend on the rate at which dye is poured in (ventilation) and rate at which water flows (blood flow)? If under steady state conditions, V is the weight of dye (in grams) entering in a short time, and Q is the volume of water (in litres) entering in the same time, the concentration of dye is given by V/Q grams per litre. In the same way, the alveolar (and blood) P_{O_2} depends

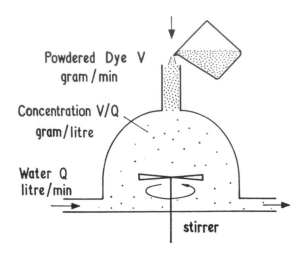

Powdered Dye V
gram / min

Concentration V/Q
gram / litre

Water Q
litre / min

stirrer

Figure 22. Model to illustrate the importance of the ventilation-perfusion ratio. Powdered dye is poured from a beaker into a stirred mixing chamber through which water flows continuously. If V is the weight of dye entering in a unit time, and Q is the volume of water entering in the same time, the concentration of dye in the mixing chamber under steady state conditions is given by V/Q.

on the *ratio* of ventilation to blood flow, or the ventilation-perfusion ratio ($\dot{V}_A/\dot{Q}$). (V stands for volume of gas, A means alveolar and the dot signifies per unit time; Q means quantity of blood and the dot means per unit time; see appendix 1 for symbols.) This ratio is the key to understanding gas exchange and it controls not only the level of P_{O_2} in alveolar gas and blood but also the P_{CO_2} and even the P_{N_2}.

The importance of the ventilation-perfusion ratio in determining regional and overall gas exchange in the lung was first recognized by two groups of workers in the United States: Rahn, Fenn and Otis and their colleagues on the one hand, and Riley and Cournand and their colleagues on the other. Most of what follows in this and the next chapter stems from these workers.

Extremes of ventilation-perfusion ratio

Suppose we take a lung unit exchanging gas under normal conditions (figure 23A). Inspired gas has a P_{O_2} of about 150 mmHg

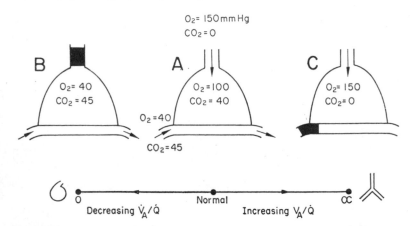

Figure 23. Extremes of ventilation-perfusion ratio. Normal gas exchange is seen in A where the balance of ventilation and blood flow is such that the alveolar $P_{O_2} = 100$ mmHg and the $P_{CO_2} = 40$ mmHg. In B, ventilation has been completely obstructed, the ventilation-perfusion ratio is nil, and the alveolar gas tensions are those of mixed venous blood (the symbol shows the right ventricle). In C, blood flow has been stopped, the ventilation-perfusion ratio is infinitely high and the alveolar gas tensions are those of inspired gas (the symbol shows the trachea). The line at the bottom shows the way the ventilation-perfusion ratio changes between these two extremes.

and a P_{CO_2} of 0; the mixed venous blood entering the lung has a P_{O_2} of about 40 mmHg and a P_{CO_2} of about 45 mmHg; the normal balance between the rates at which oxygen is added by ventilation and removed by perfusion (ventilation-perfusion ratio of about 1) gives an alveolar P_{O_2} of about 100 mmHg, and the balance between the rates at which carbon dioxide is removed by ventilation and added by perfusion gives an alveolar P_{CO_2} of about 40 mmHg; capillary blood draining from the unit has the same partial pressures as the alveolar gas.

Now suppose we gradually reduce the alveolar ventilation (but not the blood flow) by obstructing the bronchus, thus lowering the ventilation-perfusion ratio. The alveolar P_{O_2} will fall because less oxygen is being added and the P_{CO_2} will rise because less carbon dioxide is being removed. How far can these changes go? The extreme situation occurs when the ventilation is completely obstructed and we are left with a perfused but unventilated lung unit (figure 23B). The ventilation-perfusion ratio is now nil and it is clear that under these conditions the alveolar P_{O_2} and P_{CO_2} will become equal to those of the mixed venous blood, namely 40 and 45 mmHg respectively. Thus if for any reason the alveolar P_{O_2} was a little above 40 mmHg, more oxygen would be removed by the blood and, conversely, if for some reason the alveolar P_{O_2} fell below 40 mmHg, oxygen would move into the alveolar gas from the blood. (In practice, lung units which remain unventilated for long periods eventually collapse because the total gas pressure of mixed venous blood is less than atmospheric pressure but we can neglect these long term effects here.)

What happens if instead we gradually obstruct perfusion thus increasing the ventilation-perfusion ratio? Now the alveolar P_{O_2} will rise because less oxygen is being removed, and the alveolar P_{CO_2} will fall because less carbon dioxide is being added. The extreme situation occurs when perfusion is completely obstructed and the lung unit is ventilated but unperfused so that the ventilation-perfusion ratio is infinitely high (figure 23C). Now clearly the composition of alveolar gas will be identical with that of inspired gas with a P_{O_2} of 150 mmHg and a P_{CO_2} of 0, because neither the oxygen or carbon dioxide contents can be affected. In this extreme condition, we cannot talk of the gas composition of blood leaving the unit because all perfusion has stopped, but clearly the P_{O_2} and P_{CO_2} of the blood will approach nearer and nearer to those of inspired gas as perfusion is progressively reduced.

Thus the effects of extremely low and extremely high ventilation-perfusion ratios on gas exchange can be easily predicted from the compositions of the blood and gas entering the lung. In addition, we know the alveolar P_{O_2} and P_{CO_2} under normal conditions of blood flow and ventilation (figure 23A). In order to complete the picture of the effects of the ventilation-perfusion ratio on gas exchange, the oxygen-carbon dioxide diagram will be introduced because this is an invaluable aid to thinking about these relationships.

Oxygen-carbon dioxide diagram

This diagram enables us to picture the P_{O_2} and P_{CO_2} of various gas and blood samples easily and to relate them to each other. P_{O_2} is plotted horizontally and P_{CO_2} on the vertical axis (figure 24).

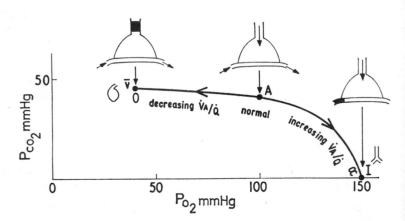

Figure 24. The oxygen-carbon dioxide diagram. The compositions of the 3 lung units of figure 23 are shown. The line joining them is known as the 'ventilation-perfusion ratio line' because it represents all the possible alveolar gas compositions as the ventilation-perfusion ratio is decreased to nil, or increased to infinity.

First locate the normal alveolar gas composition, that is a P_{O_2} of 100 mmHg and P_{CO_2} of 40 mmHg (point A on figure 24 corresponding to figure 23A). Since we are now neglecting the very small difference in partial pressures between alveolar gas and end-capillary blood (figure 5A), point A could equally well represent the gas composition of capillary blood draining from this lung unit.

Now locate the P_{O_2} and P_{CO_2} of mixed venous blood shown as $\bar{v}$ (v stands for venous and the bar above signifies 'mean' or 'mixed'). The P_{O_2} is 40 mmHg and the P_{CO_2} is 45 mmHg and as we have seen (figure 23B), this is also the alveolar gas composition of a lung unit in which ventilation has been progressively obstructed until the unit is perfused but not ventilated. Thus the line joining A to $\bar{v}$ shows how the partial pressures of alveolar gas (and blood) change as the ventilation-perfusion ratio is progressively reduced from its normal value of about 1 to zero.

Now locate the P_{O_2} and P_{CO_2} of moist inspired gas shown as I (I denotes inspired). The P_{O_2} is 150 mmHg and P_{CO_2} is 0, and this also corresponds (figure 23C) to the alveolar gas composition of a lung unit in which perfusion has been progressively reduced until the unit is ventilated but not perfused. Thus the line joining A to I shows how the composition of alveolar gas (and blood) changes as the ventilation-perfusion ratio is progressively increased from its normal value of about 1 to an infinitely high value.

The whole line $\bar{v}$ to I is called the ventilation-perfusion ratio line and its shape depends on the oxygen and carbon dioxide dissociation curves. Since it includes all possible ventilation-perfusion ratios, it represents all the possible alveolar gas partial pressures which can exist in a lung which is inspiring gas of composition I and being perfused by blood of composition $\bar{v}$. The ventilation-perfusion ratio line is therefore 'tethered' at both ends by the compositions of inspired gas and mixed venous blood so that the composition of alveolar gas (and capillary blood) can only move between these two extremes along a single line. It is not possible for example, for the lung shown in figure 24 to have an alveolus with a P_{O_2} of 50 and a P_{CO_2} of 20 as this point would clearly lie far away from the ventilation-perfusion ratio line. However the location of the line will shift if the partial pressures of mixed venous blood or inspired gas are changed. Thus if the lung of figure 24 were given a high oxygen mixture to breathe, the inspired point would move far to the right and the ventilation-perfusion

D

ratio line would become elongated. Again if the lung were hyperventilated on air for a period, the mixed venous P_{CO_2} would fall and the ventilation-perfusion ratio line would therefore be lower and flatter than in figure 24. In both instances there would be large changes in the alveolar gas composition which could be predicted from the diagram.

Regional gas tensions in the normal lung

Figure 21 shows how the ventilation-perfusion ratio increases up the normal upright lung and figure 24 shows how this ratio can be related to the alveolar gas tensions on the oxygen-carbon dioxide diagram. It now remains to locate the various levels of the normal lung on this diagram. To do this, the lung can be divided into 9 imaginary horizontal slices (corresponding to the 9 counting positions originally used to measure the distribution of blood flow shown in figure 10). The lung is assumed to be breathing air thus fixing the inspired gas point I, and reasonable values for the P_{O_2} of mixed venous blood are assumed in order to fix the mixed venous point $\bar{v}$ ($P_{O_2} = 40$ mmHg and $P_{CO_2} = 45$ mmHg in figure 25). A ventilation-perfusion ratio line can now be drawn on the oxygen-carbon dioxide diagram and the ventilation-perfusion ratio corresponding to the various points along the line calculated (see appendices for details). Knowing the ventilation-perfusion ratio of each lung slice, it is then possible to locate the position of each level of the lung on the diagram (figure 25).

It can be seen that the 9 levels of the lung from base to apex correspond to various points on the ventilation-perfusion ratio line from left to right. The ventilation-perfusion ratio increases along the line from nil at point $\bar{v}$ to an infinitely high value at point I so that the spread of the lung levels along the lung corresponds to the increasing ventilation-perfusion ratio from base to apex (figure 21). The points from the basal regions of the lung are somewhat cramped together because the ventilation-perfusion ratio changes slowly with distance up the lung in this region, but towards the apex of the lung, they spread out more.

It is now a simple matter to read off the diagram the P_{O_2} and

P_{CO_2} of alveolar gas and pulmonary capillary blood at various levels in the normal upright lung. The P_{O_2} increases up the lung at first slowly and then rapidly while the P_{CO_2} falls from base to apex. Figure 26 shows the values (top and bottom slices only for clarity) and it should be emphasised that these calculated figures and those which follow are not claimed to be exact as they are

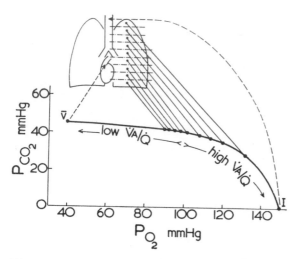

Figure 25. Oxygen-carbon dioxide diagram showing how the change in ventilation-perfusion ratio up the lung determines the regional composition of alveolar gas. The lung is divided into 9 imaginary horizontal slices each of which has its own position on the ventilation-perfusion ratio line. It can be seen that the alveolar P_{O_2} will increase up the lung in so far as the points move horizontally to the right, and that the alveolar P_{CO_2} will fall as the points move vertically downwards. Dashed lines show the composition of mixed venous (pulmonary arterial) blood and inspired (tracheal) gas.

based on several assumptions such as the composition of mixed venous blood, but the general pattern is believed to be valid. It can be seen that the P_{O_2} increases by over 40 mmHg from 89 mmHg at the base to 132 mmHg at the apex, while P_{CO_2} falls by 14 mmHg from 42 mmHg at the bottom to 28 mmHg at the top. Alveolar P_{N_2} can also be derived because the P_{O_2}, P_{CO_2} and partial pressure of water vapour must add up to 760 mmHg. Figure 26 shows that in addition to the changes in P_{O_2} and P_{CO_2}, P_{N_2} falls from the base to the apex of the upright lung. These large regional differences in gas exchange explain why the perfect lung of figure 3 had to be modified as in figure 8 to take account of ventilation-perfusion ratio inequality.

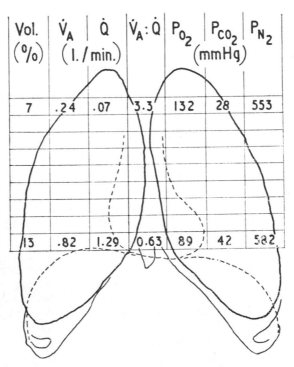

Vol. (%)	$\dot{V}_A$ (l./min.)	$\dot{Q}$	$\dot{V}_A:\dot{Q}$	P_{O_2}	P_{CO_2} (mmHg)	P_{N_2}
7	.24	.07	3.3	132	28	553
13	.82	1.29	0.63	89	42	582

Figure 26. Effects of the change in ventilation-perfusion ratio up the lung on the regional composition of alveolar gas. Values for P_{O_2} and P_{CO_2} have been read off figure 25. P_{N_2} has been obtained by difference since the total gas pressure (including water vapour) = 760 mmHg. The volumes of the lung slices, ventilation and blood flow are also shown.

Figure 26 also shows the blood flow and ventilation of each lung slice not in litres per minute percent lung volume as in figure 21, but in the simpler units of litres/minute. Thus the addition of the ventilations in the second column for all of the 9 slices gives 5.1

litres per minute which is the total alveolar ventilation, while the blood flows add up to 6 litres per minute, this being the assumed total blood flow. To put in these figures, it was necessary to assign a volume (as a percentage of the total) to each lung slice and this was done on the basis of measurements of lung shape. The regional volume of the equal thickness slices increases somewhat down the lung and is also shown in figure 26.

Regional gas exchange in the normal lung

Figure 25 shows that once the positions of the various lung levels are located on the oxygen-carbon dioxide diagram, it is easy to read off the partial pressures of oxygen and carbon dioxide in alveolar gas and pulmonary capillary blood. The diagram can also be used to derive a great deal more information about regional gas exchange. For example, it is possible to include the oxygen and carbon dioxide dissociation curves in the diagram and thus read off the oxygen and carbon dioxide contents of the end-capillary blood at different lung levels.

Figure 27A shows oxygen dissociation curves for three carbon dioxide tensions: 20, 40 and 60 mmHg. Each curve has the typical S shape with a nearly flat upper portion where there is little change in oxygen content for large changes in P_{O_2}. As the P_{CO_2} increases, the dissociation curve is shifted to the right so that for a given P_{O_2}, the blood holds less oxygen. This property enhances the unloading of oxygen in systemic capillaries and is known as the Bohr effect. Figure 27B shows carbon dioxide dissociation curves for blood of different oxygen saturations. The curves are more nearly linear than those of oxygen in the working range and the dissociation curves for decreasing oxygen saturation are displaced to the left so that for a given P_{CO_2}, the blood holds more carbon dioxide. This feature assists the loading of carbon dioxide by blood in the systemic capillaries and is often referred to as the Haldane effect.

Figure 28 shows the oxygen-carbon dioxide diagram with lines of equal oxygen content and equal carbon dioxide content superimposed on it. These lines are only a reflection of the oxygen and dioxide dissociation curves. Thus if we look at the oxygen content lines first (running upwards and to the right), it can be seen that as the P_{O_2} increases from left to right, the oxygen content increases. Similarly, pick out the carbon dioxide content lines; as the P_{CO_2} increases up the diagram, lines of increasing carbon dioxide content are encountered. The reason why the content lines are not parallel to the axes is the effect of changes in P_{CO_2} on the oxygen dissociation curve on the one hand (Bohr effect) and the effect of changes in P_{O_2} on the carbon dioxide dissociation curve on the

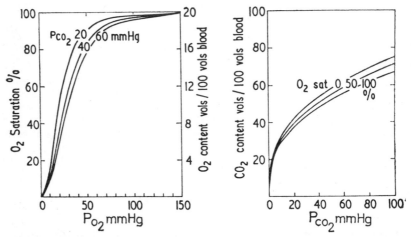

Figure 27A. Oxygen dissociation curves for blood at a P_{CO_2} of 20, 40 and 60 mmHg. Note that when the P_{O_2} is high, the dissociation curves become almost flat, and that as the P_{CO_2} is increased, the curves shift to the right. **Figure 27B.** Carbon dioxide dissociation curves for blood at different oxygen saturations. Note that these curves are straighter than the corresponding curves for oxygen and that as the oxygen saturation is increased, the curves shift to the right.

other (Haldane effect). For example, if we fix on a P_{O_2} of say 100 mmHg and move up the diagram thereby increasing the P_{CO_2}, the oxygen content falls (Bohr effect). Similarly, if we select a P_{CO_2} of say 40 mmHg and move across the diagram from left to right thus increasing the P_{O_2}, the carbon dioxide content falls (Haldane effect).

Figure 28 allows us to read off the oxygen and carbon dioxide contents of blood draining from alveoli at different levels in the upright lung. Thus the point corresponding to the bottom slice has an oxygen content between 19 and 19.5 volumes per 100 volumes of blood (actually 19.2) while the carbon dioxide content is nearly 50 volumes per cent (actually 49). The corresponding contents for the point referring to the top slice are 20 and 42 volumes per cent. In the same way, the oxygen and carbon dioxide contents of mixed venous blood can be read off the diagram: they are 14.6 and 52.4 volumes per cent respectively.

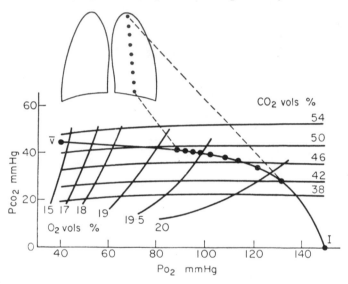

Figure 28. Oxygen-carbon dioxide diagram showing lines of equal oxygen and carbon dioxide contents. These are simply a reflection of the two sets of dissociation curves (figure 27). It can be seen that from the bottom to the top of the lung, the oxygen content of blood draining from the capillaries increases from about 19.2 to 20.0 vols/100 vols of blood, while the carbon dioxide content falls from about 49 to 42 vols/100 vols blood.

In figure 29, the oxygen and carbon dioxide contents, and oxygen saturation of blood draining from alveoli at various levels are shown. The last is calculated from the fact that 100% saturation corresponds to an oxygen content of 20 volumes per cent. Note that the percentage changes in carbon dioxide and particularly oxygen content up the lung are much less than the percentage changes in partial pressures (figure 26) because of the slopes of the dissociation curves. Thus whereas P_{O_2} changes by over 40 mmHg from the bottom to the top of the lung, the change in oxygen saturation is only 4%.

Figure 29 also shows the pH of end-capillary blood at various levels in the lung. The pH must differ because the P_{CO_2} changes up the lung (figure 26) and the standard bicarbonate content is the same. Indeed it is possible to superimpose lines of equal pH on the oxygen-carbon dioxide diagram [21] but this has not been done in figure 28 because of the confusing effect of more lines. Figure 29 shows

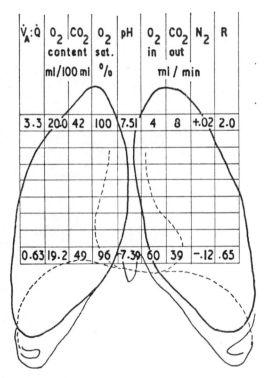

Figure 29. Effects of the change in ventilation-perfusion ratio up the lung on regional gas exchange. The oxygen and carbon dioxide contents have been read off figure 28, and oxygen saturation and pH have been calculated from these. Oxygen, carbon dioxide and nitrogen uptakes or outputs of each slice have been derived using the Fick principle. Respiratory exchange ratio R has then been computed.

that there are appreciable differences in pH from the bottom to the top of the normal lung and that the pH rises to over 7.50 at the apex.

Knowing the oxygen and carbon dioxide contents of end-capillary blood at different lung levels, we can now calculate the volumes of oxygen and carbon dioxide exchanged in the various lung slices. To do this, the oxygen and carbon dioxide contents of mixed venous blood are read off the diagram (figure 28) and the arterial-venous difference in each slice is calculated. This is then multiplied by the blood flow to give the volume of oxygen taken up and the volume of carbon dioxide given off (Fick principle). Figure 29 shows that there are very large differences in the volumes of oxygen and carbon dioxide exchanged at different levels. Thus 15 times more oxygen is taken up by the lowermost slice than the uppermost, and the corresponding figure for carbon dioxide is nearly 5. This means that at rest, the upper part of the upright lung takes little part in gas exchange, though on exercise with more blood flow to the apex (figure 16), its contribution becomes increasingly important.

An interesting aspect is the movement of nitrogen in the upright lung. Figure 26 shows that the P_{N_2} decreases from 582 to 553 mmHg from bottom to top and since under these conditions, the P_{N_2} of mixed venous blood is 575 mmHg, nitrogen will move from alveolar gas into capillary blood at the base (minus sign, figure 29) but out of the blood at the apex (plus sign). Thus there is a nitrogen cycle within the lung, the net exchange being zero since this gas is biologically inert. However the volumes of nitrogen concerned are very small.

The last column in figure 29 shows the respiratory exchange ratio, that is the volume of carbon dioxide evolved divided by the volume of oxygen absorbed in each lung slice. (It is sometimes called the respiratory quotient but this term is better reserved for the corresponding ratio for the whole organism which is determined by its metabolic requirements). Figure 29 shows that the respiratory exchange ratio increases from the base to the apex as does the ventilation-perfusion ratio (first column). In fact, the relation between respiratory exchange ratio and ventilation-perfusion ratio is a very important one and although we have reached it at the end of our tour around the oxygen-carbon dioxide diagram, it is one of the key landmarks of the diagram.

Figure 30 is an oxygen-carbon dioxide diagram with straight lines showing how the composition of inspired gas changes when various volumes of oxygen are removed from it and various volumes of carbon dioxide are added. Suppose we have a litre of inspired gas (moist air) and remove 100 ml of oxygen and replace this with 100 ml of carbon dioxide so that the respiratory exchange ratio is 1. It is easy to see that the P_{O_2} will fall by the same amount as the P_{CO_2} rises. Thus the straight line corresponding to R equals

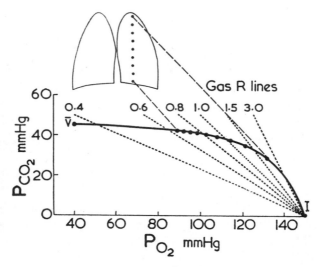

Figure 30. Oxygen-carbon dioxide diagram showing respiratory exchange ratio (R) lines for gas. These radiate from the inspired point I. It can be seen that the regional respiratory exchange ratio increases up the upright lung.

1 makes an angle of 45° with the horizontal axis. If we add less carbon dioxide than we remove oxygen (R less than 1), the P_{CO_2} will rise less than the P_{O_2} falls so the straight line will be flatter. If on the other hand, we add more carbon dioxide than we remove oxygen (R greater than 1), the P_{CO_2} will rise more than the P_{O_2} falls so the straight line will be steeper. Thus lines of equal

respiratory exchange ratio for gas form a fan which radiates out from the inspired gas point, and the R of any gas sample can be read off the diagram. Figure 30 confirms figure 29 in showing that the respiratory exchange ratio of the gas in the alveoli rises from about 0.65 to about 2 from the bottom to the top of the lung.

Figure 31 shows another set of lines radiating from the mixed

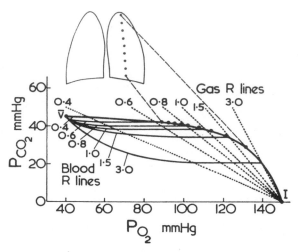

Figure 31. Oxygen-carbon dioxide diagram showing the addition of the respiratory exchange ratio (R) lines for blood. These radiate from the mixed venous point v̄ but, unlike the gas R lines, they are curved because the oxygen and carbon dioxide content lines are not straight (figure 28). Gas and blood lines for the same R intersect on the ventilation-perfusion ratio line.

venous blood point v̄. Suppose we take a sample of venous blood and add increasing volumes of oxygen to it always removing the same volume of carbon dioxide. The P_{O_2} and P_{CO_2} of the blood will then change as indicated by the line for R equals 1. In this case, the line is not straight because the relations between P_{O_2} and oxygen content, and P_{CO_2} and carbon dioxide content are not linear (figures 27 and 28). However the lines of equal respiratory exchange ratio for blood also form a fan (though this is bent) which radiates out from the mixed venous point, and once they are drawn, the R of any blood sample can be read off the diagram.

Note that any particular gas R line (say R equals 1) meets its corresponding blood R line at the ventilation-perfusion ratio line (figure 31). This must be the case because in any one lung unit in a steady state, the same volume of oxygen must be added to the blood as is removed from the alveolar gas, and vice versa for carbon dioxide. Thus the gas and blood respiratory exchange ratios must be identical. Indeed this is how the ventilation-perfusion ratio line is originally drawn (see appendix 2), that is, by joining the various points where the appropriate gas and blood R lines intersect (figure 31). We shall use these R lines extensively when we come to consider the effects of ventilation-perfusion ratio inequality on overall gas exchange (chapter 4).

At the end of this section on regional gas exchange in the normal lung it should be pointed out that the topographical distribution shown for example in figures 25 and 26 probably does not account for the whole of the ventilation-perfusion ratio inequality in the normal lung. This is partly because not all the lung is accessible to study by the radioactive gas techniques and also because there is probably some unevenness of blood flow and ventilation within a particular lung slice at the lobule or alveolar level (see section below on the diseased lung). The existence of a spread of ventilation-perfusion ratios beyond that shown in figure 25 is suggested by measurements of overall gas exchange when the lung breathes high oxygen mixtures [5, 14]. However most of the ventilation-perfusion ratio in the upright normal lung can be accounted for on a topographical basis, the evidence for this being that the calculated alveolar-arterial oxygen difference corresponds closely to that observed when normal subjects breathe air (see chapter 4).

Regional inequality of blood flow and ventilation in the abnormal lung

While it is possible to describe the pattern of ventilation-perfusion ratio inequality and therefore gas exchange for different lung units in the upright normal lung (figures 26 and 29), this can rarely be done in the diseased lung. The reason is that because of the disorganisation of the lung structure, the bulk of the ventilation-perfusion ratio inequality is at the level of small lung structures (segments, lobules or even alveoli). Thus radioactive techniques with external counters which include many cubic centimetres of lung tissue in each counting field see some sort of average of very many lung units, and the important differences in ventilation-perfusion ratio are obscured. It is true that patients with chronic obstructive lung disease for example often do have differences in blood flow and ventilation between topographical regions of both lungs and such inequalities are particularly liable to occur in the presence of bullae and cysts. However it can be shown that these regional differences in ventilation-perfusion ratio are very minor compared with the inequalities which must be present at the alveolar level.

Little is known about the mechanisms by which the disorganization of structure affects the distribution of blood flow and ventilation in the abnormal lung. It is not difficult to imagine that fibrous tissue formation for example may obstruct small blood vessels but no particular pattern of blood flow inequality has been described in diffuse interstitial fibrosis of the lung for example. More is known about the factors causing ventilatory inequality. If we regard the functional lung unit (figures 1 and 2) as an elastic chamber connected to the atmosphere by a tube (figure 32), the amount of ventilation of the unit depends on the distensibility (volume-change per unit pressure change, or compliance) of the chamber and the resistance of the tube. In figure 32, unit A has a normal distensibility and airways resistance. The rate at which its volume changes during inspiration is shown and it can be seen that the volume change is large and rapid so that it is complete before expiration for the whole lung begins (dashed line). By contrast, unit B has a low distensibility and its change of volume is rapid but small. Finally unit C has a high airways resistance so that inspiration is slow and not complete before the lung has begun to exhale. Clearly the shorter the time available for inspiration (high breathing rate), the smaller the inspired volume. Such a unit is said to have a long time constant. Thus regional inequality of ventilation will result either from alterations in local distensibility or airways resistance, and the pattern of inequality will depend on the frequency of breathing.

Another possible cause of uneven ventilation in the abnormal lung may be mentioned. It is known that inspired gas does not reach the alveoli by ordinary bulk flow but that the last milli-metre or so of distance is travelled by gaseous diffusion. In the

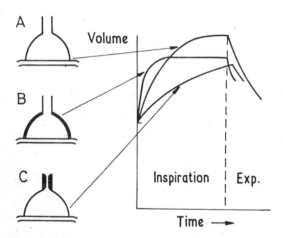

Figure 32. Effects of changes in regional airways resistance and lung distensibility (compliance) on ventilation. Unit A has a normal resistance and distensibility; note that its increase in volume is large and complete by the onset of expiration for the whole lung. Unit B has a low distensibility, its change of volume is rapid but small. Unit C has a high airways resist-ance; its change of volume is slow and is therefore not complete by the time the rest of the lung has begun to exhale (long time constant).

normal lung, the distance is so small and the diffusion rates of gases are so high that the composition of alveolar gas in the func-tional unit is uniform. Indeed this is why it is possible to regard the lung unit (figure 1) as composed of a single volume of gas of uniform composition continually undergoing gas exchange, and an airway where no gas exchange occurs (figure 33A). By contrast, the abnormal lung often contains dilated terminal airways (for example in centrilobular emphysema) and it is likely that because of the increased diffusion distances, significant non-uniformity of gas composition occurs within the alveolar volume. In this case, the simple scheme of figure 1 breaks down (figure 33B) and the resulting impairment of gas exchange can be attributed to uneven ventilation *along* the lung unit.

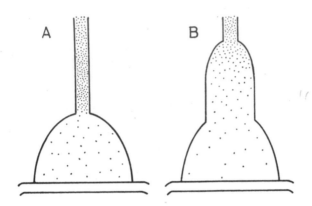

Figure 33A. Normal lung unit. Beyond the conducting airways, the alveolar gas has a uniform composition because of rapid gaseous diffusion.
Figure 33B. Lung unit with terminal airways dilated by disease. There is non-uniformity of gas composition along the lung unit because the distance to be covered by diffusion is greater.

Regional gas exchange in the abnormal lung

Although the regional inequality of blood flow and ventilation in the abnormal lung cannot be measured directly, some notion of the degree of inequality of gas exchange between different lung elements can be deduced indirectly from the observed effect of the ventilation-perfusion ratio inequality on overall gas exchange. Here we must anticipate the next chapter for a moment to point out that in spite of regional differences in P_{O_2} of over 40 mmHg in the normal lung, the net effect of this ventilation-perfusion ratio inequality on overall gas exchange is trifling. Its effect is to reduce the arterial P_{O_2} by only some 3 mmHg below that which would be present in the absence of ventilation-perfusion ratio inequality.

By contrast, the ventilation-perfusion ratio inequality caused by extensive disease of a lung may depress the arterial P_{O_2} by 50 mmHg and calculations show that the differences in ventilation-perfusion ratio which exist between lung units must be enormous. While the ventilation-perfusion ratios in the normal lung lie fairly near to the normal value particularly in the case of the low values (figure 25), in the diseased lung they may spread out along the entire ventilation-perfusion ratio line (figure 43). Indeed considerable portions of many diseased lungs must be represented by points very near to the mixed venous point on the one hand and the inspired point on the other, with the result that these lungs contain alveolar P_{O_2} and P_{CO_2} which range all the way from those of venous blood to those of inspired gas.

In general, it is impossible to divide up the diseased lung into various proportions by volume which have defined ventilation-perfusion ratios. It is because this can be done in broad terms with the normal lung that most of this chapter has been devoted to it. The normal lung thus serves as a useful foundation on which to erect the ventilation-perfusion ratio structure although as will be shown in chapter 4, ventilation-perfusion ratio inequality in the normal lung has a very small effect on overall gas exchange.

Ventilation-perfusion ratio inequality and overall gas exchange

The last chapter was concerned with the way in which differences in ventilation-perfusion ratio throughout the lung cause regional differences in P_{O_2}, P_{CO_2}, oxygen uptake, carbon dioxide output, etc. These can be dealt with systematically in the normal upright lung because the ventilation-perfusion ratio decreases in a regular manner down the lung. Although there is no such pattern in the diseased lung, even larger differences in gas exchange undoubtedly exist between different alveoli.

The present chapter is concerned with the way in which inequality of ventilation-perfusion ratios affects the overall gas exchange of the whole lung, that is, the ability of the lung to transfer oxygen from the air to the blood, and carbon dioxide in the opposite direction. We shall see that for a given lung with a certain ventilation and blood flow, the effect of introducing uneven distribution of gas and blood is to reduce the efficiency of the lung as a gas exchanger. This is the most important aspect of ventilation-perfusion ratio inequality because the success of the lung as a gas exchanger is what matters to the whole organism. For the same reason, this aspect most concerns the physician who must deal with patients whose lungs are failing. We shall again approach the subject of overall gas exchange through the normal lung because it is so orderly, and then go on to the diseased lung where the impairment of gas exchange may be very much more serious.

Impairment of gas exchange

How can we measure how efficiently the lung is doing its job of gas exchange? A convenient way of answering this question is to use the analogy of a heat exchanger (figure 34A). Suppose we have a source of hot water at 150° (Fahrenheit) from a boiler and wish to heat water which is then circulated through the radiators of a house. In the scheme shown, water returns from the radiators at a temperature of 40° and is heated to 97° in its passage through the heat exchanger which consists of a series of pipes mounted closely together in pairs (only three pairs are shown for simplicity).

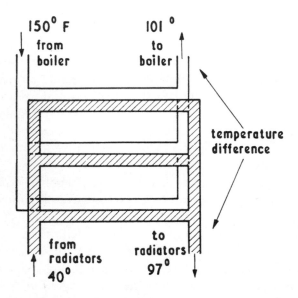

Figure 34A. Heat exchanger. Water from a boiler kept at 150°F heats water which is then circulated through the radiators of a house. If the exchanger were perfect, the temperature of the water leaving both sides of the device would be the same. Faulty heat exchange results in a fall in the temperature of the water going to the radiators, and a rise in the temperature of the water returning to the boiler. The temperature difference between these two is a useful index of impaired heat exchange.

In the process, heat is lost from the boiler water which therefore leaves the heat exchanger at a temperature of 101°. What simple criteria can we use for expressing the efficiency of the heat exchanger so that we know when it becomes faulty?

It is clear that, in general, the better the heat exchanger the higher the temperature of the water going to the radiators. However, this is not a very satisfactory criterion since, for example, by running the boiler at a higher temperature we can raise the temperature of the water going to the radiators even though the characteristics of the heat exchanger are unchanged. Again it is

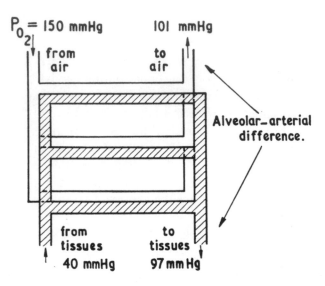

Figure 34B. Gas exchanger. Air with a P_{O_2} of 150 mm Hg circulates (actually reciprocates) on the one side of the alveolar membrane giving up oxygen to the blood. If the gas exchanger were perfect, the gas leaving it (expired alveolar gas) would have the same P_{O_2} as the arterial blood. Faulty gas exchange causes the arterial P_{O_2} to fall and the alveolar P_{O_2} to rise. The alveolar-arterial P_{O_2} difference is thus an index of impaired gas exchanged. Ventilation-perfusion ratio inequality in the normal lung causes a difference of about 4 mmHg (figure 35). Shunt and possibly diffusion factors will increase this (compare figures 3, 6, 7, 8).

clear that, in general, the better the heat exchanger, the lower the temperature of the water returning to the boiler (the more heat has been given up) but again this measurement by itself could be misleading. A more useful measurement than either temperature separately would be the difference between the temperatures of the two effluent streams. Thus if the design of the heat exchanger were very good, the difference between the temperatures would be very small, while if some fault developed such as some of the pipes on the boiler or radiator side becoming narrowed by boiler scale, heat exchange would become less efficient and an increasing temperature difference between the two outflowing streams would develop.

By analogy, the lung apposes air and blood so that gas can exchange (figure 34B shows typical values for oxygen). In fact, alveolar ventilation is reciprocating, not continuous as shown in the figure but this is immaterial in the present context. Inefficient gas exchange will show up both as a fall in arterial P_{O_2} and a rise in alveolar P_{O_2}, but a better criterion than either of these alone is the difference between the two. Thus in a perfect gas exchanger the alveolar-arterial oxygen (and carbon dioxide) difference would be nil (figure 3), while as the lung became faulty, the alveolar-arterial gas differences would increase. In the normal lung, the alveolar-arterial oxygen difference due to ventilation-perfusion ratio inequality is about 4 mmHg as shown in figure 34B but this may increase many fold as the gas exchange of the lung is impaired by disease.

The heat exchanger analogy points to the value and limitations of alveolar-arterial differences as simple criteria of the efficiency of gas exchange. It is clear that a true figure of merit would take into account the amount of heat transferred, the temperatures of the incoming streams of water etc. However, in practice, alveolar-arterial differences are often useful guides to the impairment of gas exchange partly because the amounts of gas transferred are approximately fixed by the metabolic requirements, and the composition of inspired gas and mixed venous blood vary little at rest. Nevertheless one of the advantages of the more refined criteria of impaired gas exchange which we shall meet later such as the size of the physiologic dead space and the amount of venous admixture is that these indices are less affected by the other factors mentioned above.

Alveolar-arterial differences

The difference in partial pressure between alveolar gas and arterial blood is the simplest index of impaired gas exchange and it is worth calculating the alveolar-arterial differences which will develop in the normal lung as a result of the uneven blood flow and ventilation shown in figures 21 and 26. Figure 35 shows the main features of the calculation for oxygen; the calculations for carbon

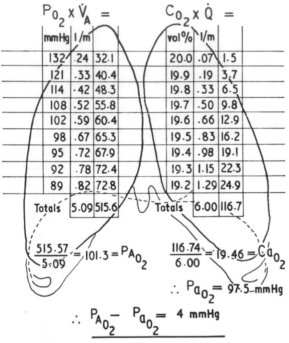

$$P_{O_2} \times \dot{V}_A = \qquad C_{O_2} \times \dot{Q} =$$

mmHg	l/m		vol%	l/m	
132	.24	32.1	20.0	.07	1.5
121	.33	40.4	19.9	.19	3.7
114	.42	48.3	19.8	.33	6.5
108	.52	55.8	19.7	.50	9.8
102	.59	60.4	19.6	.66	12.9
98	.67	65.3	19.5	.83	16.2
95	.72	67.9	19.4	.98	19.1
92	.78	72.4	19.3	1.15	22.3
89	.82	72.8	19.2	1.29	24.9
Totals	5.09	515.6	Totals	6.00	116.7

$$\frac{515.57}{5.09} = 101.3 = P_{A_{O_2}} \qquad \frac{116.74}{6.00} = 19.46 = C_{a_{O_2}}$$

$$\therefore P_{a_{O_2}} = 97.5 \text{ mmHg}$$

$$\therefore P_{A_{O_2}} - P_{a_{O_2}} = 4 \text{ mmHg}$$

Figure 35. Calculation of the alveolar-arterial difference for P_{O_2} in the normal lung. To find the mixed alveolar oxygen tension ($P_{A_{O_2}}$) the ventilation ($\dot{V}_A$) of each slice is multiplied by the regional P_{O_2} (figures 25 and 26), the products are summed and divided by the total ventilation. To find the arterial oxygen tension ($P_{a_{O_2}}$), the blood flow ($\dot{Q}$) of each slice is multiplied by the regional oxygen content of the blood (figures 28 and 29), the products are summed and divided by the total blood flow. This arterial oxygen content ($C_{a_{O_2}}$) is then converted into a P_{O_2}. It can be seen that the ventilation-perfusion ratio inequality results in an alveolar-arterial P_{O_2} difference of 4 mm Hg. (Some small inconsistencies occur in the above table because not all the decimal places are shown.)

dioxide and nitrogen are similar. To find the mixed alveolar oxygen tension (P_{AO_2}), the alveolar P_{O_2} is multiplied by the alveolar ventilation ($\dot{V}_A$) of each slice since the contribution of a slice to the total expired volume is proportional to its own ventilation. The products are then summed and divided by the total ventilation (5.09 litres/min) to give the mixed expired alveolar P_{O_2} (101 mmHg). Similarly, to find the mixed capillary (arterial) oxygen tension (Pa_{O_2}), the oxygen content of the blood leaving each slice (figure 29) is multiplied by its blood flow ($\dot{Q}$) and the products summed (figure 35). (We must always add contents, not partial pressures, when dealing with blood; summing partial pressures in gas is only valid because content and partial pressure are proportional.) When the sum is divided by the total blood flow (6 litres/min), we have the oxygen content of arterial blood (Ca_{O_2}; 19.46 vols/100 vols blood). This is now converted into P_{O_2} by referring to the oxygen-carbon dioxide diagram of figure 28 giving a value of 97 mmHg. Thus the alveolar-arterial difference is 4 mmHg. Similar calculations for carbon dioxide and nitrogen give arterial-alveolar differences of 1 and 3 mmHg respectively (in both cases, the arterial value is higher than the alveolar).

These calculations help to show why alveolar-arterial differences develop. Figure 35 shows that the lower slices of the lung are much more important in determining the arterial blood composition than are the upper slices because the base of the lung is much better perfused than the apex. Since the lower slices have lower oxygen contents than the upper slices the result is that the arterial P_{O_2} is depressed becaused it is loaded with less well oxygenated blood. By contrast, the difference of ventilation between the upper and lower slices is much less marked than for blood flow with the result that the mixed alveolar P_{O_2} is more nearly an average of the individual slices. Thus a disproportionate amount of blood from the lower slices enters the arterial blood compared with the amount of alveolar gas they contribute (figure 36). An alveolar-arterial difference is therefore inevitable.

There is a second reason for the alveolar-arterial oxygen difference which is not so apparent from figure 35. Figure 37 shows three groups of alveoli in a mythical patient in whom disease has so interfered with the distribution of blood flow and ventilation that the left hand group has 10 times as much blood flow but only one-tenth of the ventilation as the middle (normal) group, while the figures are reversed for the right hand group. Blood draining from the group on the left will have a low oxygen content because the ventilation-perfusion ratio is only $\frac{1}{10}$ (from an oxygen-carbon dioxide diagram like that of figure 28, an oxygen content

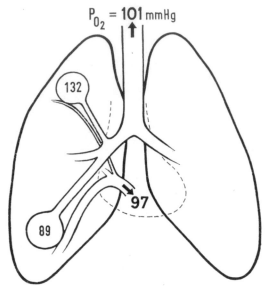

Figure 36. Development of the alveolar-arterial difference for P_{O_2} in the normal lung. Relative sizes of the bronchi and pulmonary veins to the upper and lower zones indicate their relative ventilations and blood flows. Only two groups of alveoli are shown corresponding to those in the uppermost and lowermost slices in figure 25. Mixed pulmonary venous blood has a slightly low P_{O_2} (97 mmHg) because most of the blood comes from the base of the lung which has a low P_{O_2} (89 mmHg). In mixed alveolar gas a greater proportion comes from the apex of the lung which has a higher P_{O_2} (132 mm Hg). An alveolar-arterial difference of 4 mmHg results from this ventilation-perfusion ratio inequality. (From *The Lancet*.)

of 16 vols/100 vols blood can be calculated for an alveolus with this ventilation-perfusion ratio). However blood draining from the group on the right will hardly have a higher content than blood coming from normal lung which is over 95% saturated. Thus the mixed blood must have a low oxygen content. This second reason for the alveolar-arterial oxygen difference thus depends on the peculiar shape of the oxygen dissociation curve and does not apply to carbon dioxide or nitrogen.

A striking feature of the alveolar-arterial differences caused by ventilation-perfusion ratio inequality in the normal lung is that they are so small. We have seen earlier that in spite of regional differences of alveolar P_{O_2} of over 40 mmHg, the alveolar-arterial oxygen difference is only 4 mmHg which is

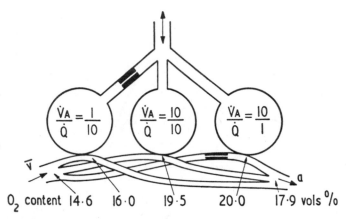

$$\frac{\dot{V}_A}{\dot{Q}} = \frac{1}{10} \qquad \frac{\dot{V}_A}{\dot{Q}} = \frac{10}{10} \qquad \frac{\dot{V}_A}{\dot{Q}} = \frac{10}{1}$$

O_2 content   14·6   16·0   19·5   20·0   17·9 vols %

Figure 37. Diagram to show an additional cause for the alveolar-arterial difference for oxygen. Three groups of alveoli with very low (left hand), normal and very high (right hand) ventilation-perfusion ratios are shown. Note that although the oxygen content of the blood draining from the alveoli on the left is much reduced (16 vols %) the blood draining from the alveoli on the right is only slightly above normal (20.0 compared with 19.5 vols %). This is because of the shape of the oxygen dissociation curve (figure 27). Combined with the effect of the greater contribution to the arterial blood of the alveoli on the left, the result is a considerable lowering of the arterial oxygen content (17.9 vols %.)

almost immeasurably small. In the case of carbon dioxide, regional differences of 14 mmHg exist and yet the arterial-alveolar difference is only 1 mmHg, while for nitrogen the difference between uppermost and lowermost slices is 29 mmHg but the arterial-alveolar difference is only 3 mmHg. By contrast, the corresponding differences between alveolar gas and arterial blood in the diseased lung may be very large—over 50 mmHg for example for oxygen.

It is important to be clear about the sense in which 'alveolar' has been used so far in the phrase 'alveolar-arterial difference'. We have been referring to the partial pressure of *mixed expired* alveolar gas, that is, all the gas exhaled from the lung excluding that which comes from the conducting airways which is anatomic dead space and takes no part in gas exchange (figure 1). In the analogy of the heat exchanger of figure 34A, this corresponds to the temperature of the mixed boiler water as it left the heat exchanger. Alveolar gas is thus analogous to arterial blood which is the mixed effluent from the other side of the alveolar membrane, the only difference being that there is no anatomic dead space on the blood side.

A great practical limitation of the use of mixed alveolar-arterial differences defined in this way is that it is often impossible to measure the alveolar gas partial pressures in the presence of disease. The reason is that in many abnormal lungs (for example, in chronic airways obstruction, and pulmonary fibrosis), alveoli with a high ventilation-perfusion ratio tend to empty first and those with a low ventilation-perfusion ratio empty last. Since the gas exhaled in the first part of expiration is contaminated by anatomic dead space gas, this must be discarded, and the result is that any subsequent alveolar sample is not representative of expired alveolar gas. This difficulty does not arise in normal lungs or in some diseased lungs, for example, following pulmonary emboli, where alveoli empty together and an end-tidal sample is representative of mixed expired alveolar gas. (An end-tidal sample is one collected at the end of a normal expiration which should be large enough to wash out the anatomic dead space.) The practical value of alveolar-arterial differences is discussed in chapter 5.

Ideal alveolar gas

The mixed alveolar-arterial difference is the simplest index of impaired gas exchange due to ventilation-perfusion ratio inequality but it cannot always be measured, and when it can it tells us nothing about the pattern of uneven distribution which is present. For this, we must introduce the notion of ideal alveolar gas and here again, the oxygen-carbon dioxide diagram is indispensable.

Figure 38 shows figure 25 with the addition of the alveolar (A) and arterial (a) points which are derived as in figure 35. Because

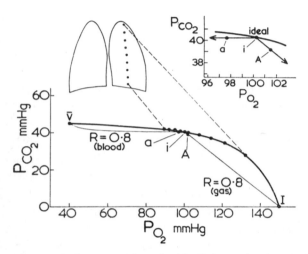

Figure 38. Oxygen-carbon dioxide diagram showing the ideal (i) alveolar (A) and arterial (a) points. The ideal point is at the intersection of the gas and blood R lines corresponding to the respiratory exchange ratio of the whole lung. Ventilation-perfusion ratio inequality causes displacement of the alveolar point along the gas R line (dead space), and the displacement of the arterial point along the blood R line (venous admixture). The inset shows that the resulting alveolar-arterial difference in the normal lung is about 4 mmHg for oxygen and 1 mmHg for carbon dioxide.

they lie close together, an inset shows the relationships more clearly. The alveolar-arterial difference for oxygen is the horizontal distance between the two points and the carbon dioxide difference is the vertical separation. Now is there any way of predicting how these points will move as the ventilation-perfusion ratio inequality becomes more severe? The answer to this lies in the respiratory exchange ratio lines (R lines) which were discussed in figures 30 and 31. A moment's thought will show that no matter how severe the ventilation-perfusion ratio inequality and therefore how widely separated are the alveolar and arterial points, they *must* lie on their respective gas and blood R lines because the respiratory exchange ratio of both gas and blood is determined by the metabolism of the body. This is simply another way of saying that the amount of carbon dioxide added to alveolar gas by the blood, divided by the amount of oxygen removed from it (gas R), is determined *for* the lung *by* the body in a steady state. Likewise the amount of carbon dioxide lost by the capillary blood divided by the volume of oxygen gained by it is also fixed. In figure 38, both points are situated on R lines of 0.8. If blood flow and ventilation were more unevenly distributed in this lung, the alveolar and arterial points would move further away from each other along their R lines. Conversely, if the amount of ventilation-perfusion ratio inequality were reduced, the two points would move closer together, still on their R lines.

What is the significance of the point of intersection of the gas and blood R lines for 0.8? This point must denote the composition of alveolar gas *and* arterial blood in a lung with *no* ventilation-perfusion ratio inequality when this lung is exchanging gas at the same R as the actual lung. This point is known as the ideal point (i).

We now see more clearly what happens to the composition of alveolar gas and arterial blood as ventilation-perfusion ratio inequality is imposed on a lung. Both points move away from the ideal point along their respective R lines. Thus we have separated the alveolar-arterial difference into two components one being represented by the movement of the alveolar point away from the ideal point, and the other by the movement of the arterial point away from the ideal point. The first is said to be due to 'alveolar dead space', and the second the consequence of 'venous admixture'.

Alveolar and physiologic dead space

Let us look more closely at the movement of the alveolar point along the gas R line (figure 39). Suppose we take 100 ml of ideal gas (which in this lung has the composition P_{O_2} = 100 mmHg,

$P_{CO_2} = 40$ mmHg) and mix it with 100 ml of inspired gas ($P_{O_2} = 150$ mmHg; $P_{CO_2} = 0$). The mixture will have a P_{O_2} halfway between 100 and 150 mmHg and a P_{CO_2} halfway between 40 and 0 mmHg, so that its composition will be represented by a point exactly halfway between the ideal and inspired points, that is halfway down the gas R line (point B). Similarly a mixture of one part of ideal gas with 3 parts of inspired gas (total four parts) will

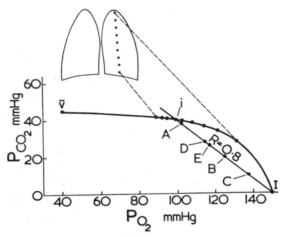

Figure 39. Oxygen-carbon dioxide diagram showing dead space effects. The addition of increasing amounts of dead space causes the alveolar point to move further and further along the gas R line from the ideal (i) towards the inspired gas point (I). A mixture of 50% dead space and 50% ideal alveolar gas results in a composition halfway along the line at point B. In the normal lung, ventilation-perfusion ratio inequality is equivalent to the addition of 3% dead space to the ideal alveolar gas and the composition of the *mixed alveolar* gas is shown at A. *Mixed expired* gas contains anatomic dead space gas which moves its composition further down the line to E. For further explanation, see text.

be represented by a point three-quarters of the way down the gas R line (point C). Thus increasing dilution of the ideal gas with inspired gas is represented by progressive movement of the point down the gas R line. Now the anatomic dead space contains inspired gas at the end of inspiration so that we could just as easily say that increasing addition of *dead space gas* to ideal gas is represented by movement down the gas R line. Thus we could say that the alveolar point moved away from the ideal point just *as if* dead space were added to ideal gas. In other words, we can attribute that part of the alveolar-arterial difference caused by movement of the alveolar point to the addition of dead space gas. In the normal lung (figure 38) the movement of the alveolar point is equivalent to adding 3% of dead space to the ideal alveolar gas. This figure is obtained by dividing the distance i to A, by the total distance i to I, and multiplying by 100.

It is important to emphasise that the alveolar gas does not contain any real dead space gas from the conducting airways. However the term is not such a fanciful one as it may appear at first sight. Consider what alveoli have been responsible for the movement of the alveolar point down the gas R line. They are the alveoli in the lung slices which lie to the right of the ideal point along the ventilation-perfusion ratio line, that is the alveoli of the upper 5 slices which have high ventilation-perfusion ratios and therefore a high P_{O_2} and low P_{CO_2} (figures 25 and 26). Furthermore, it is clearly the slices which lie furthest away from the ideal point which have the greatest effect on the alveolar point (neglecting for a moment the fact that the volume contribution of these slices to expired alveolar gas is less). It is as if the alveolar point were pulled along the gas R line by alveoli with high ventilation-perfusion ratios. Indeed, an alveolus with an infinitely high ventilation-perfusion ratio has no blood flow at all (figure 24) and functionally is indistinguishable from anatomic dead space which itself is ventilated but unperfused.

Thus it is perfectly reasonable to attribute that part of the alveolar-arterial difference caused by movement of the alveolar point, to dead space admixture. However to distinguish this dead space from anatomic dead space, it is called *alveolar dead space* since it originates in the alveoli. Another way of referring to the movement of the alveolar point is to attribute it to '*wasted ventilation*' just as that portion of the inspired tidal volume which remains in the anatomic dead space is wasted from the point of view of gas exchange. Whatever term is used, the true cause of the movement is the presence in the lung of alveoli with ventilation-perfusion ratios above that corresponding to the ideal point.

Let us take a last look at the gas R line. We have seen that the addition of anatomic dead space gas to ideal gas will move the composition down the line. This is just what happens if we collect all the gas exhaled through the lips using a mouthpiece and valve box; each 350 ml or so of alveolar gas is mixed with 150 ml or so of anatomic dead space gas (figure 2). The composition of the resulting mixture will be represented by a point $150/500 = 3/10$ of the way from i to I down the gas R line (point D). Now if alveolar gas has a composition represented by A because it contains alveolar dead space, the mixed expired gas will be represented by a point further down the R line (point E = expired).

The mixed expired point E is of great practical importance because this gas can be easily collected and its composition measured (see chapter 5). As a consequence, it is convenient to refer to the movement of the point all the way from the ideal point i to the expired point E as due to the addition of *physiologic dead space*. This term therefore includes the effects of alveolar dead space (distance i to A) and anatomic dead space (distance A to E). Physiologic dead space is thus made up of contributions from alveoli which have ventilation-perfusion ratios exceeding that of ideal alveoli, and the volume of gas contained in the anatomic dead space.

Venous admixture

Venous admixture, or the addition of mixed venous blood to arterial blood is by analogy the 'alveolar dead space' of blood. There are two small differences between the behaviour of blood and gas; one is that there is no 'anatomic dead space' on the blood side because blood flows in only one direction through the lung, and the other is that movement of the arterial point along the blood R line is not as regular as that of gas along its R line because of the non-linear blood dissociation curves. However the principles for blood and gas are very similar.

Suppose we take 100 ml of ideal capillary blood (i) and add 100 ml of mixed venous blood (v̄) (figure 40). The oxygen and carbon dioxide *contents* of the mixture must lie halfway between those of i and v̄ at point b. Note that because the oxygen and carbon dioxide content lines are not regularly spaced on the oxygen-carbon dioxide diagram (figure 28) because the dissociation curves are not linear (figure 27), the P_{O_2} and P_{CO_2} of b are

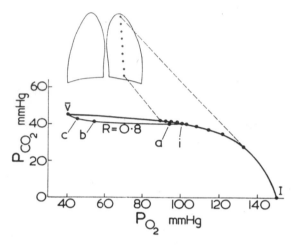

Figure 40. Oxygen-carbon dioxide diagram showing venous admixture effects. The addition of increasing amounts of venous blood causes the arterial point to move further and further along the blood R line from the ideal (i) towards the mixed venous blood (v̄) point. A mixture of 50% venous blood and 50% ideal capillary blood results in a composition represented by point b which has oxygen and carbon dioxide *contents* halfway between those of points i and v̄ (figure 28). In the normal lung, ventilation-perfusion ratio inequality is equivalent to the admixture of about 1% of venous blood with the ideal blood and the composition of the mixed pulmonary venous blood is shown at a. For further explanation, see text.

not halfway between those of i and v̄. Now suppose we add 300 ml of mixed venous blood to 100 ml of ideal blood; the resulting mixture will have a composition represented by c which has oxygen and carbon dioxide *contents* three-quarters of the way along the blood R line from i. Thus increasing addition of venous blood to ideal blood progressively moves the composition of the mixture out along the blood R line from i to v̄.

It follows that the movement of the arterial point from i to a as a result of the ventilation-perfusion ratio inequality in the lung can be attributed to venous admixture just as the movement of the alveolar point from i to A can be attributed to the admixture of alveolar dead space. Again note that the movement from i to a does not necessarily mean that any of the pulmonary capillaries are really contributing venous blood, but that the arterial blood composition changes *as if* venous blood were being added. This time the alveoli responsible for the displacement of the arterial point are those which lie to the left of the ideal point on the ventilation-perfusion ratio line and have low ventilation-perfusion ratios (lower 4 slices in figure 25). The further away these alveoli are from the ideal ventilation-perfusion ratio, the more will they pull the arterial point away from the ideal point. Indeed if any alveoli are actually unventilated but perfused (figure 24), the blood leaving them will be unchanged venous blood so that their whole contribution will be venous admixture. This blood is wasted from the point of view of gas exchange and sometimes the movement of the arterial point away from the ideal is attributed to '*wasted blood flow*'.

While there is no blood space which is analogous to the anatomic dead space because blood flow is in only one direction, a diseased lung may contain direct connections between the pulmonary arteries and veins such as fistulae which will contribute 'anatomic' venous admixture. These true shunts (figure 7) will move the arterial point along the blood R line thus contributing to the alveolar-arterial differences just as will alveoli with low ventilation-perfusion ratios. Ways of distinguishing these two causes of hypoxaemia are discussed in chapter 5. In the normal lung (figure 38), the movement of the arterial point is equivalent to adding about 1% of venous blood to ideal capillary blood. This figure is obtained by dividing the difference in oxygen contents between i and a, by the difference in oxygen contents between i and v̄, and multiplying by 100.

In practice, the displacement of the arterial point away from the ideal point is sometimes expressed simply as the horizontal distance between the two points, that is the (ideal alveolar)-arterial oxygen difference. Often the word 'ideal' is omitted so that this alveolar-arterial difference (or A-a 'gradient') should be distinguished from the (mixed expired alveolar)-arterial difference which we have been discussing here. Generally the context prevents any confusion though sometimes it is necessary to precede the word 'alveolar' by either 'mixed' or 'ideal'.

We have seen how to divide the simple (mixed) alveolar-arterial difference into one part due to alveolar dead space which is caused by alveoli with high ventilation-perfusion ratios, and another part attributable to venous admixture which is caused by alveoli with low ventilation-perfusion ratios. Apart from the added information about the pattern of ventilation-perfusion ratio inequality in the lung which this approach gives, it has the additional advantage that the calculated alveolar dead space and venous admixture are not so affected by changes in the composition of inspired gas and mixed venous blood as is the simple alveolar-arterial difference. Thus the new criteria of impairment of gas exchange are more useful figures of merit for the lung.

Special patterns of ventilation-perfusion ratio inequality

It might be thought that with our increasing understanding of the way in which ventilation-perfusion ratio inequality affects gas exchange, it should be possible to recognize various patterns of ventilation-perfusion inequality in different lung diseases. In fact this is seldom possible as yet. There are however a few conditions which are associated with particular patterns.

Pulmonary hypotension

One of the simplest patterns of ventilation-perfusion ratio inequality is that of progressive non-perfusion of the upper parts of the lung. We have seen that blood rises up the lung only to the level at which pulmonary arterial pressure equals alveolar

F

pressure (figures 12 and 14), so that if the arterial pressure is reduced or the alveolar pressure increased, alveoli at the apex will be unperfused. There is evidence that this pattern may occur in haemorrhage, positive-pressure breathing, anaesthesia and exposure to increased acceleration.

Figure 41 shows the gas exchange of an upright lung in which arterial pressure is less than alveolar pressure in the uppermost four slices. Since these slices are unperfused, their ventilation-perfusion ratio is infinitely high so the points representing their

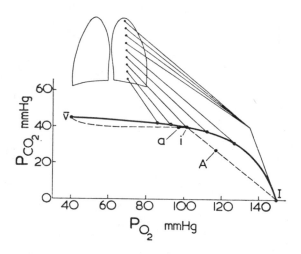

Figure 41. Gas exchange in a lung with its upper zone unperfused. Ventilation is normally distributed. The positions on the ventilation-perfusion ratio line of the points representing the lung slices should be compared with those in the normal lung (figure 25). Now the upper 4 slices have an infinitely high ventilation-perfusion ratio and their points have moved to the inspired gas point I. This results in large alveolar-arterial differences for oxygen and carbon dioxide (20 and 13 mmHg respectively). The alveolar dead space (distance i to A) is much increased now being 32% of the alveolar tidal volume. The diagram emphasises how alveoli with very high ventilation-perfusion ratios 'pull' the alveolar point down along the gas R line (compare figure 38). By contrast, venous admixture (distance i to a) is almost unchanged at 2% of the total pulmonary blood flow. This pattern may be found in pulmonary hypotension due to haemorrhage, anaesthesia, and in positive pressure breathing.

alveolar P_{O_2} and P_{CO_2} are located at the inspired point (I). The positions of the other six points are determined by their respective ventilation-perfusion ratios. In this lung, the total ventilation and therefore the overall ventilation-perfusion ratio have been increased to keep the respiratory exchange ratio and arterial P_{CO_2} at the normal levels. Figure 41 also shows the arterial (a), Alveolar (A) and ideal (i) points. The alveolar point has been displaced from the ideal by alveolar dead space, and the arterial point has been moved by venous admixture.

It can be seen that the result of this pattern of ventilation-perfusion ratio inequality has been to create a large alveolar dead space but virtually no additional venous admixture compared with the normal lung (figure 38). The alveolar dead space is now 32% of the total alveolar tidal volume while the venous admixture component is almost unchanged being 2% of the total pulmonary blood flow. This is not unexpected since the four unperfused slices are functionally indistinguishable from anatomic dead space while none of the lung has an unduly low ventilation-perfusion ratio which would contribute much additional venous admixture. There is now considerable ventilation-perfusion ratio inequality in that the ratio varies from 0.59 to infinity rather than 0.63 to 3.3 as in the normal lung (figures 21 and 26) but in spite of this, the arterial P_{O_2} and P_{CO_2} are normal. The alveolar arterial differences for these gases have been increased to 20 and 13 mmHg respectively; the alveolar ventilation was raised by three-quarters of its original value.

This type of impaired gas exchange occurs in acute haemorrhage, and also positive pressure ventilation. The former has been shown to reduce the pulmonary arterial pressure, and in positive pressure breathing, the alveolar pressure rises more than the arterial pressure so that the net result in both is unperfused alveoli at the top of the lung. Exposure to increased vertical acceleration also results in unperfused alveoli at the apex but the resulting gas exchange is complicated by reduced ventilation at the base of the lung (see below). Pulmonary embolism is another condition characterised by a large alveolar dead space but little venous admixture though here the unperfused alveoli are not regularly disposed.

Reduced ventilation at lung bases

Another common pattern of impaired gas exchange is characterised by areas at the bottom of the lung which have very low
ventilation-perfusion ratios. This pattern occurs in the lung
during prolonged anaesthesia, particularly in patients who are
unable to take deep breaths because of pain. Other causes include
partial obstruction of the lower zone airways by bronchial secretions or inhaled liquids. Figure 42 shows an upright human lung
in which the two lowermost slices are normally perfused but
virtually unventilated. As a result, their ventilation-perfusion
ratios are almost nil and they make a minimal contribution to
gas exchange. The figure shows the development of alveolar-
arterial differences of 53 and 6 mmHg for oxygen and carbon
dioxide respectively. The venous admixture component is greatly
increased to the equivalent of 42 % of the total pulmonary blood
flow but the alveolar dead space is only 3 % which is the same as
in the normal lung (figure 38). The pattern contrasts with the gas
exchange of pulmonary hypotension (figure 41) where the char-
acteristic change is in the alveolar dead space and venous admixture is hardly affected. In practice, this pattern is always associated
with completely unventilated alveoli which are functionally identical to right to left shunts (figure 7). Alveoli with low ventilation-
perfusion ratios can be distinguished from those which are totally
unventilated by giving the patient oxygen to breathe (see page 100).

A useful rule which emerges from these two patterns is that
in general, inequality of blood flow causes increased alveolar dead
space, and inequality of ventilation causes increased venous
admixture. The reason for this is that for groups of alveoli to have
any large influence on the movement of the alveolar or arterial
points away from the ideal point, they must either have very high
or very low ventilation-perfusion ratios. In the normal lung for
example (figure 38), although the lowermost and (particularly)
the uppermost slices lie some distance away from the ideal point,
the resulting displacement of the arterial and alveolar points is
very small with the result that the calculated dead space and venous admixture are only 3 and 1% respectively. In practice, in
order to obtain the very high or very low ventilation-perfusion

ratios necessary to cause clinically significant dead space or venous admixture, either blood flow or ventilation must be greatly reduced in some area (figures 41 and 42). By contrast, an *increased* blood flow through one lung zone resulting, say, from vascular obstruction in another zone will not sufficiently lower the ventilation-perfusion ratio to cause significant venous admixture. For the same

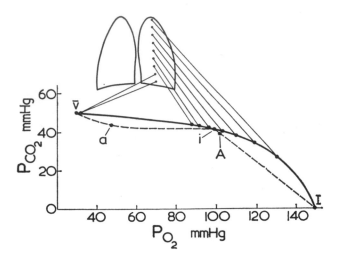

Figure 42. Gas exchange in a lung with its lower zone very poorly venti-lated. Blood flow is normally distributed. Compare the locations of the lung slices on the ventilation-perfusion ratio line with those in the normal lung (figures 25 and 38) Now the lower 2 slices have very low ventilation-perfusion ratios and their points have moved very close to the mixed venous blood point v̄. This again results (compare figure 41) in large alveolar-arterial differences for oxygen and carbon dioxide (53 and 6 mmHg respectively). However now the venous admixture component (distance i to a) is much increased being 42% of the total pulmonary blood flow. This emphasises how alveoli with very low ventilation-perfusion ratios 'pull' the arterial point along the blood R line. By contrast, dead space (distance i to A) is virtually unchanged compared with the normal lung being 3% of the alveolar tidal volume. This pattern may be found in patients who lie still for long periods because of loss of consciousness or pain, or when secretions partially block the lower zone airways. In practice, this pattern is always associated with true shunts through completely unventilated alveoli. Note that the P_{O_2} of mixed venous blood has been reduced by 5 mmHg and the P_{CO_2} increased by 5 mmHg compared with figures 25 and 38.

reason, an increase of ventilation in a normally perfused area contributes very little to alveolar dead space in practice. Hence the rule of thumb: inequality of blood flow causes dead space, while inequality of ventilation causes venous admixture.

Exposure to high acceleration

This results in a combination of the two previous patterns (figure 43). When the lung is accelerated upwards, the apex is unperfused causing a large physiological dead space. This may be looked

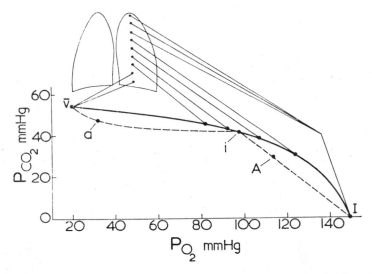

Figure 43. Gas exchange in a lung with its upper zone unperfused and its lower zone very poorly ventilated. Now only the middle 4 slices are contributing significantly to gas exchange. Enormous alveolar-arterial differences for oxygen and carbon dioxide have developed (80 and 20 mmHg respectively). Alveolar dead space (distance i to A) is now 29% of the alveolar tidal volume, and venous admixture (distance i to a) is 55% of the total pulmonary blood flow. This pattern may be found during rapid upward acceleration of the lung when the increased weight of the blood results in an unperfused apex, and the increased weight of the lung interferes with ventilation at the base. However the chief importance of this type of impaired gas exchange with large dead spaces and venous admixtures, is that it occurs in many generalized lung diseases, though not on a topographical basis.

upon as a consequence of the increased weight of the blood and is analogous to perfusing the lungs with mercury. Just as the weight of the blood is increased, so is the weight of the lung with the result that the intrapleural pressure at the base rises and the airways tend to close. (The same mechanism is responsible for the non-ventilation of the base of the lung when its volume is small, figure 20B.) Thus we are left with a lung which is unperfused at the apex and virtually unventilated at the base; only the mid zones are exchanging gas to a significant degree. Figure 43 shows the development of both a large alveolar dead space (equivalent to 29% of the alveolar tidal volume) and a large venous admixture component (equivalent to 55% of the total pulmonary blood flow). The alveolar-arterial differences are 80 mmHg for oxygen and 20 mmHg for carbon dioxide.

This pattern has been described not because exposure to high accelerations is a common hazard but because this large spread of ventilation-perfusion ratios occurs in many generalized lung diseases. In these however, there is no systematic change down the lung and there is as yet no way of locating the positions of various volumes of the lung on the ventilation-perfusion ratio line. All we can say is that in chronic obstructive lung disease, for example, large alveolar dead spaces and venous admixture effects are commonly found and these must reflect a great mismatch of ventilation and perfusion. Defining the various patterns of ventilation-perfusion ratio inequality must wait until more refined analytical techniques are available.

Ventilation-perfusion ratio inequality as a barrier to gas exchange

One way of looking at ventilation-perfusion ratio inequality is as a barrier to gas exchange in that it interferes with the lung's ability to take up oxygen and put out carbon dioxide. It is not a mechanical barrier in the sense that thickening of the alveolar membrane may impede the diffusion of oxygen through it (figures 5 and 6) but it is nevertheless a barrier which must be overcome by some 'compensatory' change in the behaviour of the lung if the same quantities of gas are to be transferred. It would be impossible for example for a lung which developed ventilation-perfusion ratio inequality to transfer oxygen and carbon dioxide at the same partial pressures with the same overall ventilation and blood flow as it did previously.

This can be shown by taking a model lung with its blood flow and ventilation evenly distributed, and calculating its oxygen uptake and carbon dioxide output. For figure 44, the same total blood flow and ventilation, and the same composition of mixed venous blood were assumed as in figure 25. Now what is the effect on overall gas exchange of suddenly imposing the normal pattern of ventilation-perfusion ratio inequality on this model lung? Figure 44 shows that the result is to decrease the volumes of both oxygen and carbon dioxide transferred by the lung; oxygen uptake

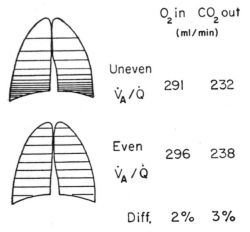

	O_2 in	CO_2 out
	(ml/min)	
Uneven $\dot{V}_A/\dot{Q}$	291	232
Even $\dot{V}_A/\dot{Q}$	296	238
Diff.	2%	3%

Figure 44. Ventilation-perfusion ratio inequality as a barrier to gas exchange. The amounts of oxygen and carbon-dioxide transferred by a model lung are compared before and after the imposition of ventilation-perfusion ratio inequality. Both models have the same overall ventilation and blood flow and are supplied with the same venous blood and inspired air. The pattern of ventilation-perfusion ratio inequality is that found in the normal lung (figure 21). Note that the result of the uneven distribution has been to reduce the efficiency of the lung as a gas exchanger so that oxygen uptake and carbon dioxide output fall by 2 and 3 per cent respectively. (From BRITISH POSTGRADUATE MEDICAL FEDERATION (1966), *The Scientific Basis of Medicine*, London, Athlone Press.)

falls by 2% and carbon dioxide output by 3%. These are small changes it is true, but the principle is important: the lung with ventilation-perfusion inequality loses efficiency as a gas exchanger. The small impairment in the case of the normal pattern of ventilation-perfusion inequality reflects the small alveolar dead space or wasted ventilation, and the small venous admixture or wasted blood flow in the normal lung. However, just as these indices of ventilation-perfusion ratio inequality may become very large in the diseased lung, so the lung's inefficiency as a gas exchanger becomes more marked.

It is worth looking at the way in which a lung copes with the imposition of ventilation-perfusion ratio inequality. If we take an imaginary lung and suddenly mismatch its ventilation and blood flow, alveolar-arterial differences will immediately develop so that the alveolar P_{O_2} will rise and the P_{CO_2} fall; in the arterial blood, the P_{O_2} will fall and the P_{CO_2} rise (figure 38). Since the arterial P_{O_2} falls, the arterio-venous oxygen difference will be reduced and unless overall blood flow increases, the oxygen uptake will fall (Fick principle). This may happen temporarily, but in a steady state the volumes of oxygen and carbon dioxide transferred by the lung are determined for it by the metabolic demands of the body so that some other solution must be found. What generally occurs is that the P_{O_2} of mixed venous blood also falls thus restoring the arterio-venous oxygen difference and therefore the oxygen uptake.

The problem in the case of carbon dioxide is similar. When ventilation-perfusion ratio inequality is imposed on the lung, the arterial P_{CO_2} rises and the alveolar P_{CO_2} falls (figure 38). However the carbon dioxide output of the lung must be restored and a possible solution is that the arterial P_{CO_2} (and mixed venous P_{CO_2}) rise. But we now have to take account of a factor outside the lung, that is the respiratory centre which responds to any tendency for arterial P_{CO_2} to rise by increasing the respiratory drive. Thus the usual result is that the arterial P_{CO_2} (and mixed venous P_{CO_2}) return to their former level but ventilation to the alveoli is increased. The additional ventilation is 'wasted' on the alveolar dead space. To summarise the usual final solution, the result of imposing ventilation-perfusion ratio inequality is to lower the arterial P_{O_2} (and mixed venous P_{O_2}) but to maintain the arterial P_{CO_2} at its former level, while the ventilation to the alveoli is increased.

These manoeuvrings become clear when oxygen-carbon dioxide diagrams for diseased lungs are drawn (figures 41 to 43). For example in figure 41, the unperfused upper zone causes a large alveolar dead space and it was found that alveolar ventilation had to be increased by three-quarters of its original value to return the carbon dioxide output of this lung to the previous level. An alternative strategy would have been to allow the arterial (and mixed venous) P_{CO_2} to rise but this is unrealistic because the normal respiratory centre would generally not allow it. Again in figure 42, the large venous admixture effect lowers the arterial P_{O_2} and therefore the arterial-venous oxygen difference, with the result that the oxygen uptake falls. This could have been returned to its previous level by increasing the cardiac output but a more realistic solution is to reduce the P_{O_2} of mixed venous blood and leave total blood flow constant. In figure 43 it was necessary both to increase ventilation and to lower the mixed venous P_{O_2}.

These possible solutions have been discussed at some length to emphasise that ventilation-perfusion ratio inequality interferes with the transfer of both oxygen *and* carbon dioxide. The former is usually obvious enough because the patient is either cyanosed or the arterial P_{O_2} is reduced, but it is less easy to see that carbon dioxide transfer has been affected when the arterial P_{CO_2} is normal. The fact is that ventilation-perfusion ratio inequality is a barrier to carbon dioxide output but by raising the ventilation to the alveoli, the lung can often return the arterial P_{CO_2} to its normal level.

One way of emphasising the impairment of carbon dioxide exchange which results from ventilation-perfusion inequality is to calculate the rise in arterial P_{CO_2} which would have occurred if the patient had not increased the ventilation to his alveoli. Suppose a patient with chronic obstructive lung disease is found to have a normal arterial P_{CO_2} of 40 mmHg but an alveolar dead space of one-third of his total alveolar tidal volume (that is, a physiologic dead space/tidal volume of about 50%). Calculations show that this patient might have had an arterial P_{CO_2} of about 60 mmHg if he had not increased the ventilation to his alveoli in response to his respiratory centre drive (the figure depends on the pattern of ventilation-perfusion ratio inequality). Alternatively we can say that if the same patient with his arterial P_{CO_2} of 40 mmHg suddenly had his ventilation-perfusion ratio inequality abolished while the ventilation to his alveoli remained unchanged, his arterial P_{CO_2} might fall to the vicinity of 25 mmHg. Such calculations emphasise the great importance of ventilation-perfusion ratio inequality in interfering with carbon dioxide elimination as well as oxygen uptake. The only reason why its effect on carbon dioxide transfer is not so generally appreciated is that the respiratory centre is so efficient in holding the arterial P_{CO_2} constant by raising the ventilation.

Carbon dioxide retention

Some patients with ventilation-perfusion ratio inequality develop carbon dioxide retention and since high concentrations of carbon dioxide in the blood are narcotic, this condition is potentially dangerous. Why does the arterial P_{CO_2} rise in these patients? Progressive lung disease (perhaps aggravated by an acute infection) causes increasing mismatch of blood flow and ventilation with larger alveolar-arterial differences and greater impairment of carbon dioxide excretion. For a time the body is able to keep the rising arterial P_{CO_2} in check by increasing the ventilation to the alveoli, but the work of breathing in these patients is usually high because of the increased airways resistance so that eventually a compromise is reached and the arterial and alveolar P_{CO_2} are allowed to rise. This has the advantage that more carbon dioxide is put out for the same ventilation so that it can be looked upon as a compensatory mechanism, albeit a hazardous one. As the ventilation-perfusion ratio inequality becomes worse, the tendency is for the arterial P_{CO_2} to rise further. This is particularly likely to occur if the hypoxic respiratory drive is abolished by giving the patient pure oxygen to breathe.

Patients with ventilation-perfusion ratio inequality and carbon dioxide retention are sometimes said to be 'hypoventilating'. This term is used by people who define the adequacy or otherwise of alveolar ventilation by whether it maintains a normal arterial P_{CO_2}. Thus 'hypoventilation' in this context really simply means an increased arterial P_{CO_2}. 'Alveolar ventilation' in this context does not refer to all the gas entering the lung alveoli but is related to 'ideal alveolar' and excludes alveolar dead space gas. In this monograph, the term 'alveolar' has been used to refer to all the lung, excluding the conducting airways which contain anatomic dead space (figure 1). True hypoventilation was discussed on page 6 and carbon dioxide retention caused by hypoventilation is shown in figure 51.

An important feature of carbon dioxide retention caused by ventilation-perfusion ratio inequality is that it can usually be temporarily relieved by the patient voluntarily increasing his ventilation, although occasionally the work of breathing is so high that the additional effort produces more carbon dioxide than the extra ventilation excretes. In these instances, assisted ventilation by means of a respirator will reduce the arterial P_{CO_2}. The fact that increasing the ventilation relieves the carbon dioxide retention is sometimes regarded as evidence that its cause is 'hypoventilation'. However the root cause of the carbon dioxide retention is ventilation-perfusion ratio inequality although its effects on the arterial P_{CO_2} can be overcome by increasing the ventilation to the alveoli.

Mechanisms reducing ventilation-perfusion ratio inequality

It is clear that there may be gross inequality of blood flow and ventilation in a lung and yet no ventilation-perfusion ratio inequality if the distributions of blood flow and ventilation are identical. While this extreme situation is never observed, there is evidence that some matching of blood flow and ventilatory inequality does occur in the diseased lung.

There are probably several reasons for this. The first is that many disease processes reduce both blood flow and ventilation in a given area by their destruction of the regional architecture.

Localized fibrosis, for example, interferes both with perfusion and ventilation, and the same is generally true of cysts and localized infection such as an abscess. There is no need to look for compensating mechanisms in these instances; one has only to cut through an area of dense fibrosis to appreciate that normal blood flow and ventilation would be impossible.

However there are active mechanisms which probably operate to reduce the deleterious effects of uneven blood flow and ventilation on gas exchange. Since the initial observation that alveolar hypoxia increases the pulmonary artery pressure in the cat, there have been many demonstrations of vasoconstriction and the movement of blood flow away from hypoxic areas of the lung in man and in other animals. The precise mechanism is still disputed but it appears to be a local response since it occurs in the isolated denervated lung. In man, there is evidence that the alveolar P_{O_2} must be reduced to low levels—less than 50 mmHg for example—but as figure 43 shows, many of the alveoli in a severely diseased lung are likely to have a P_{O_2} below this. It is thought that this vasoconstriction of hypoxic areas may contribute to the high pulmonary vascular resistance of obstructive lung disease.

Another mechanism which may play a part is the increased airways resistance which follows the obstruction of blood flow to a region of lung. This is apparently caused by the fall in P_{CO_2} in the area which increases the resistance of the small airways. There have been several direct or indirect demonstrations of this mechanism in various species. Again it apparently only operates at a low P_{CO_2} but a severely diseased lung certainly contains alveoli with a very low P_{CO_2} (figure 43).

Such mechanisms could greatly improve the gas exchange of a lung in which blood flow and ventilation were disturbed. In the first place, they would tend to restore the ventilation-perfusion ratios of abnormal areas towards the normal value. In addition, by reducing the blood flow or ventilation to these abnormal areas, their contribution to overall gas exchange would be limited and the diverted blood flow and ventilation would go to more useful regions of the lung.

The beneficial results of these changes are shown in figure 45, where these compensatory mechanisms have been allowed to operate on the grossly abnormal lung of figure 43. In figure 43, the blood flow to the upper three zones was abolished and the ventilation to the lower two zones was drastically reduced. Apart from these changes, however, both blood flow and ventilation maintained their normal pattern with the result that the unperfused upper part of the lung received an appreciable ventilation and the virtually unventilated lower zone received a large blood flow. In figure 45, ventilation to the unperfused apex has been greatly diminished so that although the ventilation-perfusion ratio is still infinitely high (there is no blood flow), the contribution of this part of the lung has been severely restricted. Likewise, the blood flow to the almost unventilated base has been greatly reduced, and in this instance the increase in ventilation-perfusion ratio is evident from the movement of the points along the ventilation-perfusion ratio line.

It can be seen that a striking improvement in overall gas exchange followed these changes. The alveolar-arterial differences for oxygen and carbon dioxide have almost vanished so reducing the alveolar dead space and venous admixture to negligible values. Gas exchange is actually better than in the normal lung of figure 38 because virtually only the middle four slices are functioning, and these have little inequality of blood flow or ventilation. In this figure, the 'compensatory' changes in blood flow and ventilation have been carried to an extreme extent to show how great an improvement in gas exchange is theoretically possible by these mechanisms. Clearly all intermediate stages between the grossly impaired gas exchange of figure 43 and the excellent function of figure 45 are possible depending on how closely ventilation and blood flow are matched in the abnormal areas at the apex and base of the lung. The result shown emphasizes that it is not only the spread or range of ventilation-perfusion ratios which affects gas exchange but equally the ventilation and blood flow contributions of the abnormal areas. Again it should be emphasized that although the deranged pattern of figure 43 was introduced by referring to exposure to high acceleration, its importance is that this type of impaired gas exchange with large dead spaces and venous admixtures occurs in most generalised lung diseases, though not on the regional basis shown in the figure.

What is the evidence that some matching of blood flow and ventilation occurs in chronic lung diseases? The next chapter describes how a measure of the inequality of blood flow and ventilation in the lung can be obtained by the analysis of single ex-

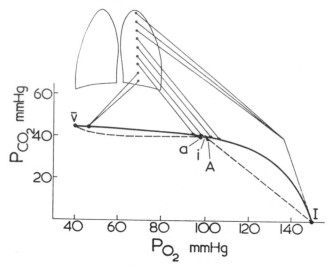

Figure 45. Effects of gas exchange in the lung of figure 43 when the ventilation to the unperfused upper zone is greatly reduced and the blood flow to the virtually unventilated lower zone is also decreased. Note that the alveolar-arterial differences for oxygen and carbon dioxide have now almost vanished; alveolar dead space and venous admixture have become negligibly small. Indeed gas exchange is better than in the normal lung of figure 38 because virtually only the middle four slices are functioning, and these have little inequality of blood flow or ventilation. This figure emphasizes that it is not only the spread of ventilation-perfusion ratios which affects gas exchange but equally the ventilation and blood flow contributions of the abnormal areas.

pirations. Such measurements have shown that poorly ventilated alveoli empty last during expiration and that, in many patients, these poorly ventilated alveoli are poorly perfused. This has been found in chronic obstructive bronchitis and emphysema, diffuse interstitial fibrosis, sarcoidosis, and other chronic lung diseases. The same conclusion has been drawn from the two compartment analysis of the lung which is also described in chapter 5. Here the lung is divided into two theoretical compartments on the basis of ventilation rates, and again it is found that the poorly ventilated alveoli are poorly perfused. Most of these studies have been made in patients thought to have pulmonary emphysema. It is noteworthy that even in the normal upright lung, the deleterious effects of a very low blood flow at the apex are countered by the reduced ventilation in this area, although there is no evidence that blood flow and ventilation affect one another in this case.

What is alveolar gas?

It is worth looking at the ways in which the term 'alveolar gas' is used. In this monograph, the term has been applied to all the gas in the lung excluding that in the connecting airways, that is the anatomic dead space (figure 1). It is clear that alveolar gas does not have a single composition in the normal lung (figures 8 and 26), far less in the abnormal lung (figures 41, 42 and 43). Furthermore, even if there was no ventilation-perfusion ratio inequality within the lung, the fact that ventilation is discontinuous (breath by breath) must result in some variation of composition during the respiratory cycle. Thus at the end of inspiration the P_{O_2} of alveolar gas is higher than the mean, and it slowly falls as oxygen is removed until the next inspiration begins. The fluctuations are kept small by the large volume of alveolar gas compared with the inspired volume. Nevertheless changes in P_{O_2} and P_{CO_2} of about 3 and 2 mmHg respectively have been calculated to occur with normal breathing at rest. On exercise, the fluctuations are greater.

'Alveolar gas' is used in other ways as well. We have seen that 'ideal alveolar' refers to the composition of alveolar gas which the lung *would* have if there was no ventilation-perfusion ratio inequality and the lung continued to exchange gas at the same respiratory exchange ratio. 'Alveolar' is sometimes used to denote end-tidal, that is, the gas exhaled at the end of a normal expiration. In normal subjects this approximates to mixed expired alveolar gas at rest, but in patients with lung disease this may not be so. The reason is that well ventilated alveoli empty early and poorly ventilated alveoli empty late in expiration so that a spot sample cannot be truly representative of all. The same objection can be levelled at the post-dead space 'alveolar' sample. In some respiratory function tests (for example, the measurement of diffusing capacity by the single breath method) the gas exhaled after the anatomic dead space has been washed out is collected. In abnormal lungs, such a sample may be very different from mixed expired alveolar gas.

There is no objection to the use of the term alveolar in these different ways if it is accurately defined each time. However it is clear that there is no single answer to the question: what is alveolar gas, since its composition varies throughout the lung and in time, and, in any case, this cannot be accurately determined in many abnormal lungs. This is the reason why the notion of ideal alveolar gas is so valuable in practice.

G

Chapter 5

Methods of measuring ventilation-perfusion ratio inequality

This chapter deals with the principles of various methods of measuring ventilation-perfusion ratio inequality. For practical details, the original publications should be consulted.

Alveolar-arterial differences

The difference is partial pressures between mixed expired alveolar gas and arterial blood constitutes the simplest index of ventilation-perfusion ratio inequality but unfortunately the method can only be used in relatively few diseased states. The alveolar P_{O_2} and P_{CO_2} are preferably obtained with rapid gas analysers. They may be measured simultaneously with a respiratory mass spectrometer, or separately with an infrared carbon dioxide analyser and a rapid thermal conductivity or paramagnetic oxygen analyser. Figure 46 shows the changes in expired P_{CO_2} measured at the lips when a normal subject exhales. First pure anatomic dead space is exhaled, then increasing amounts of alveolar gas as the dead space is gradually washed out, and finally pure alveolar gas is sampled, the so-called alveolar plateau. It has been shown that a tidal volume of 750 ml is required to be reasonably certain that pure alveolar gas has been obtained. End-tidal gas samples can also be collected with mechanical samplers and analysed later. However continuous sampling by a rapid gas analyser is preferable because it is then easier to see whether the dead space has been completely washed out and also whether the subject is in a steady state.

Arterial blood should be collected simultaneously and its

P_{O_2} and P_{CO_2} measured using appropriate electrodes. It is advisable that both gas and blood analysers are calibrated using the same gas mixtures and tonometered blood.

An increased alveolar-arterial P_{O_2} difference may be due to right to left shunts (figure 7) or possibly to diffusion limitations

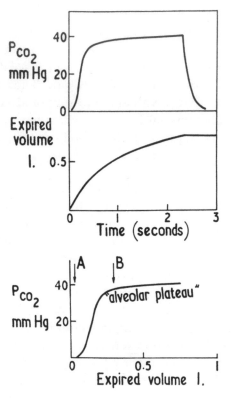

Figure 46. Diagram of tracings from a rapid carbon dioxide analyser and a flow meter sampling at the lips. In the bottom graph, expired P_{CO_2} has been plotted against expired volume. Up to arrow A, pure anatomic dead space was exhaled and the P_{CO_2} was zero. Between arrows A and B, increasing amounts of alveolar gas were added, and after B the 'alveolar plateau' is shown. In order to use end-tidal gas for the measurement of alveolar-arterial differences, it is essential that the sample is from the alveolar plateau so that there is no contamination by gas from the anatomic dead space.

(figures 5 and 6) as well as to ventilation-perfusion ratio inequality. If the last is the cause, the P_{O_2} difference alone gives no information about the pattern of ventilation-perfusion ratio inequality because both alveolar dead space and venous admixture contribute to it (figures 38, 39 and 40).

By contrast, the alveolar-arterial P_{CO_2} difference is almost solely caused by alveolar dead space. This is because the blood R lines along which the arterial point moves due to venous admixture are almost horizontal at their right hand ends (figures 31 and 40) so that large amounts of venous admixture hardly affect the arterial P_{CO_2} at all. On the other hand, alveolar dead space does reduce the alveolar P_{CO_2} considerably (figure 39). Thus the alveolar-arterial P_{CO_2} difference is a valuable measure of alveolar dead space. Increased alveolar-arterial P_{CO_2} differences have been demonstrated in pulmonary embolism, haemorrhage, positive pressure breathing, anaesthesia and exposure to increased acceleration.

Unfortunately, the use of an end-tidal sample of alveolar gas is only valid if all alveoli empty together during expiration. In many diseases such as chronic bronchitis and emphysema, and pulmonary fibrosis, alveoli with a high ventilation-perfusion ratio empty early and those with a low ventilation-perfusion ratio tend to empty late so that a post-dead space sample is not representative of the whole expired alveolar gas. Under these circumstances, the alveolar-arterial differences cannot be determined so that the application of this simple technique is limited. An end-tidal sample can also be misleading on exercise when the alveolar gas P_{O_2} and P_{CO_2} fluctuate so much during the respiratory cycle owing to the high oxygen uptake and carbon dioxide output.

Ideal alveolar gas, physiologic dead space and venous admixture

Many aspects of the analysis of the alveolar-arterial difference using the notion of ideal alveoli as introduced by Riley and Cournand [6, 23, 24, 25] were dealt with in chapter 4 (figures 38 to 45). It was shown there that not only does this approach give more information than the simple alveolar-arterial differences but it has the great advantage that it is applicable to any diseased lung. In this section, some of the more practical details of its use will be discussed.

First how is the composition of ideal alveolar gas determined? We know that the ideal point lies at the intersection of the gas and blood R lines on the oxygen-carbon dioxide diagram (figure 47). How can we find this point knowing the composition of inspired gas, mixed expired gas, and arterial blood? It is clear that the ideal

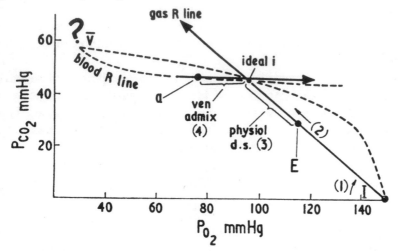

Figure 47. Analysis of Riley and Cournand using the notion of ideal gas. In practice, only 3 points are known: inspired gas I, mixed expired gas E, and arterial blood a. The problem is to find the physiologic dead space and the venous admixture component. This is done in 4 steps using 4 equations (see text) which are illustrated by this oxygen-carbon dioxide diagram. Step 1 argues that the ideal point must lie on the gas R line, and equation (1) derives the slope of this line from the inspired and mixed expired gas points. Step 2 argues that the ideal P_{CO_2} must be very close to the known arterial P_{CO_2} because the blood R line is so flat in this region; equation (2) therefore tells us to go up the gas R line until we come to the arterial P_{CO_2}. This point is then (very nearly) the ideal point. Step 3 says that the ratio of physiologic dead space to tidal volume is the distance i to E divided by the distance i to I and equation (3) calculates this. Step 4 says that the ratio of venous admixture to total blood flow is the oxygen content difference between i and a, divided by the oxygen content difference between i and v̄. The latter is not known but can be assumed with sufficient accuracy for clinical purposes. Equation (4) calculates this.

point must lie on a straight line (the gas R line) which passes through the inspired and mixed expired points. We also know that the blood R line passes through the arterial point though we cannot fix the line because we do not know the position of the mixed venous point. However, the blood R line is so nearly horizontal near the ideal point (figure 31) because of the shape of the blood dissociation curves (figure 28) that the error in using the arterial P_{CO_2} for the ideal P_{CO_2} is generally very small and this is what is done. Knowing the position of the ideal point, the distances to the expired gas and arterial blood points are known and thus the physiologic dead space and venous admixture can be determined.

In practice expired gas is collected over a period of several minutes together with arterial blood over part of this time. It is not necessary to draw an oxygen-carbon dioxide diagram. The respiratory exchange ratio R may be calculated from the expired P_{O_2}, P_{CO_2} and P_{N_2} using the expression

$$R = \frac{P_{E_{CO_2}}}{P_{I_{O_2}} \cdot \dfrac{P_{E_{N_2}}}{P_{I_{N_2}}} - P_{E_{O_2}}} \qquad (1)$$

where E and I refer to expired and inspired respectively (see appendix 1 for further explanation of symbols). In words, this equation simply derives the slope of the gas R line knowing the vertical and horizontal distances of the expired point from the inspired point (figure 47). The ideal alveolar P_{O_2} is then calculated from the alveolar gas equation:

$$P_{A_{O_2}} = P_{I_{O_2}} - \frac{P_{a_{CO_2}}}{R} + \left[\frac{0.209 . P_{a_{CO_2}} (1 - R)}{R} \right] \qquad (2)$$

This equation says that to find the ideal P_{O_2}, start at the inspired point (first term on the right hand side) and move along the R line until the arterial (ideal) P_{CO_2} is reached (second term on the right). The term in square brackets is a correcting factor of small magnitude. Thus the two equations which look rather daunting initially are only doing with symbols what we have been doing all the time graphically.

Having located the ideal point, how do we express the ventilation-perfusion ratio inequality in terms of dead space and venous admixture? We saw in chapter 4 (figure 39) that the displacement of the expired point from the ideal point is caused by both alveolar and anatomic dead space and that the combined effects of these two can be attributed to physiologic dead space. If a quarter of the tidal volume is physiologic dead space, the expired point will lie one quarter of the way along the line joining ideal and inspired points, and as the physiologic dead space increases, so the expired point will move further towards the inspired point. Thus the ratio of physiologic dead space to tidal volume equals the distance i to E divided by the distance i to I. In symbols,

$$\frac{V_D}{V_T} = \frac{Pa_{CO_2} - PE_{CO_2}}{Pa_{CO_2} - PI_{CO_2}}$$

where V_T and V_D are the tidal and dead space volumes respectively. Since $PI_{CO_2} = 0$ in air, this becomes

$$\frac{V_D}{V_T} = \frac{Pa_{CO_2} - PE_{CO_2}}{Pa_{CO_2}} \tag{3}$$

In practice, this value for dead space will contain some valve box dead space which should be subtracted. The upper limit for the physiologic dead space/tidal volume ratio is about 0.3 at rest and rather less on exercise. Higher values may be found in elderly subjects.

The calculation of the venous admixture component which moves the arterial point away from the ideal point is made in a similar way. As shown in chapter 4 (figure 40), if one quarter of the blood leaving the lung is venous admixture, the arterial point will move one quarter of oxygen *content* difference between the ideal and venous points (figure 28), and as the venous admixture component increases, so the arterial point will move further towards the venous point. Thus the ratio of venous admixture to total blood flow equals the oxygen content difference between i and a divided by the content difference between i and $\bar{v}$. In symbols,

$$\frac{\dot{Q}va}{\dot{Q}t} = \frac{Ci_{O_2} - Ca_{O_2}}{Ci_{O_2} - C\bar{v}_{O_2}}$$

where $\dot{Q}va$ and $\dot{Q}t$ are the venous admixture and total pulmonary blood flows respectively and C_{O_2} refers to the various oxygen contents. In practice, the oxygen content of venous blood is not often known but it can be estimated without serious error in the calculated venous admixture. At rest, it is usual to use a figure of 5 volumes of oxygen/100 volumes of blood for the denominator in the equation above and the venous admixture measured in this way should be less than 5%. Increases in both physiologic dead space and venous admixture are usually found in patients with ventilation-perfusion ratio inequality though predominance of one or the other occurs in some conditions (see chapter 4).

Alveolar-arterial nitrogen difference

The two methods of measuring ventilation-perfusion ratio inequality considered so far are the ones in general use but there are several procedures which show promise for the future. One is that based on the measurement of the partial pressure difference for nitrogen between arterial blood and alveolar gas. We have seen that ventilation-perfusion ratio inequality causes regional differences in P_{N_2} (figure 26) in that alveoli with a low ventilation-perfusion ratio have a high P_{N_2} and vice versa. As a result, an alveolar-arterial difference develops for nitrogen just as it does for oxygen and carbon dioxide (figure 48). A valuable feature of the nitrogen difference is that it is unaffected by right to left shunts (figure 7) because the P_{N_2} of mixed venous blood and arterial blood are identical (there is no metabolism of dissolved nitrogen in the tissues). In addition, it can be shown that an alveolar-end capillary difference for nitrogen is very unlikely so that impaired diffusion will not cause an alveolar-arterial difference (compare oxygen, figure 5). Thus the alveolar-arterial difference for P_{N_2} is affected only by ventilation-perfusion ratio inequality [4].

Figure 48 shows that the lines of equal P_{N_2} on an oxygen-carbon dioxide diagram are almost parallel to the normal gas R line (they are actually parallel to the line for $R = 1$). Thus as the alveolar point moves down the gas R line, the P_{N_2} hardly changes

so that it is little affected by physiologic dead space (figure 48).
The alveolar-arterial difference for P_{N_2} is therefore chiefly a
measure of venous admixture by contrast with the alveolar-
arterial P_{CO_2} difference which chiefly measures physiologic dead
space. It also follows from this that it is generally unnecessary to
measure alveolar P_{N_2} because this can be assumed with little
error. The P_{N_2} of arterial blood is obtained by gas chroma-
tography. It has been suggested that the P_{N_2} of urine reflects the
P_{N_2} of blood [13] but the validity of this is not certain.

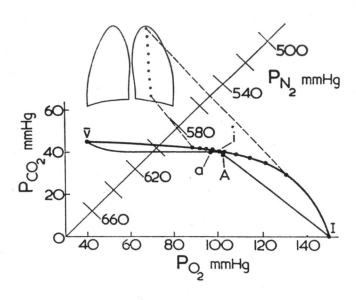

Figure 48. Oxygen-carbon dioxide diagram showing how the P_{N_2}
changes. The lines of equal P_{N_2} run diagonally across the diagram and are
parallel to the R gas line for R = 1 (figure 30). It can be seen that the P_{N_2}
decreases up the upright lung. Note also that increasing amounts of dead
space will little affect the alveolar P_{N_2} because as the alveolar point moves
down the gas R line, the P_{N_2} hardly changes. Thus the alveolar-arterial
difference for nitrogen is chiefly determined by alveoli with a low ventilation-perfusion ratio so that it is largely a measure of venous admixture. The
nitrogen scale is not strictly accurate for blood but nearly so.

Two compartment analysis

One way of measuring the inequality of ventilation in a lung is to record the gradual washout of nitrogen when a subject is given pure oxygen to breathe. If all the alveoli were evenly ventilated, nitrogen would be washed out strictly exponentially so that a plot of end-tidal P_{N_2} against the number of breaths would be a straight line on a semi-logarithmic scale. In practice, diseased lungs often produce a curved line which can be split into two (sometimes more) exponentials which correspond to two populations of alveoli, one ventilated fast and the other slowly. It is not suggested that all the alveoli really have one of these two ventilation rates; rather this is a convenient model which fits the data reasonably well.

This multibreath washout analysis has been combined with measurements of arterial oxygen saturation and oxygen consumption to determine the perfusion of each ventilated compartment [2]. It has been shown, for example, that an emphysematous lung may behave as if nine tenths of the total ventilation and one half of the total blood flow go to one quarter of the volume of the lung, whereas the other three-quarters of the volume receives only one tenth of the ventilation and the other half of the blood flow. Thus such a lung apparently has small volume of fast-ventilating alveoli with a high ventilation-perfusion ratio, and a large volume of slow-ventilating alveoli with a low ventilation-perfusion ratio. Similar results were found using an extension of this method in which radioactive krypton was injected into the venous side of the circulation and evolved into alveolar gas (compare the radioactive xenon technique, figure 9B) from which it was eliminated at a rate determined by the ventilation.

Both these techniques surmount the problem of dealing with millions of alveoli each having their own ventilation and blood flow, by regarding them as belonging to only two groups—one fast ventilated and the other slowly ventilated. In some respects, this procedure is analogous to the ideal alveolar gas analysis where the complicated effects of ventilation-perfusion ratio inequality on gas exchange are simply attributed to a certain proportion of wasted ventilation (physiologic dead space) on the one hand and a certain proportion of wasted blood flow (venous admixture) on the other. Indeed some people refer to ideal alveolar analysis as a three compartment system: ideal alveoli, dead space and venous admixture.

The analysis of the lung into two compartments, one ventilated fast and the other slowly, means that there is inevitably a spread of ventilation-perfusion ratios within each of the two groups of alveoli. Thus the difference in 'mean' ventilation-perfusion ratio between the two compartments gives no indication of the true variation within the lung. The model simply states that if the lung were composed of two uniformly ventilated compartments, their perfusions must be such and such if the arterial oxygen saturation or krypton washout rate are as measured.

Single breath analysis

It was shown in chapter 3 that differences in ventilation-perfusion ratio are associated with differences in the local respiratory exchange ratio (figures 29 and 31). Thus as the ventilation-perfusion ratio changes from 3.3 to 0.63 from the top to the bottom of the normal upright lung, R changes from 2.0 to 0.65. We have also seen that in most diseased lungs, alveoli with a high ventilation-perfusion ratio tend to empty early in expiration and those with a low ventilation-perfusion ratio tend to empty late. This fact which so limits the value of the simple alveolar-arterial difference as an index of ventilation-perfusion ratio inequality makes it possible to assess this inequality by measuring the change in respiratory exchange ratio during a single expiration [27].

In practice, expired gas is analysed with a respiratory mass spectrometer or some other rapid gas analyser and the change in R during expiration is calculated from the expired P_{O_2} and P_{CO_2} (figure 49) being careful to correct for the presence of water vapour. It is convenient to analyse the expiration following a single inspiration of an argon mixture containing 21% oxygen because this allows the inequality of ventilation to be derived from the change in expired argon [28], and the calculation of R is not affected. In this way indices of both ventilation and ventilation-perfusion ratio inequality can be obtained from a single breath. A convenient portion of the expiration to analyse is the 500 ml following the exhalation of 750 ml to clear the anatomic dead space which affects the index of ventilation (though not the ventilation-perfusion ratio). It is necessary to assume values for the composition of venous blood (as in the derivation of venous admixture)

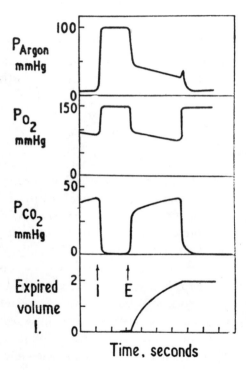

Figure 49. Derivation of ventilation, ventilation-perfusion ratio and perfusion inequality from the analysis of a single expiration. Diagram of a mass spectrometer tracing showing the changes at the lips during an expiration following a single inspiration of a mixture of about 15% argon, 20.9% oxygen and the rest nitrogen. I and E indicate the start of inspiration and expiration respectively. From the oxygen and carbon dioxide tracings, the change in expired R can be calculated to given an index of ventilation-perfusion ratio inequality. The slope of the argon tracing gives an index of ventilation inequality. By combining these two, an index of perfusion inequality can be derived.

but this can be done with little resulting error. Finally, from the inequalities of ventilation and ventilation-perfusion ratio, it is possible to derive the inequality of perfusion which must be present.

All these indices of inequality are minimal values in that in so far as alveoli having different ventilation-perfusion ratios (for example) empty together, so existing differences will be concealed. Also it is theoretically possible that a change in emptying pattern of the alveoli could reduce the observed degree of inequality of ventilation-perfusion ratio although the mismatch of blood flow and ventilation remained unchanged. However in practice it is unusual not to find an abnormal change in expired R in patients who have ventilation-perfusion inequality.

Inert gas elimination

It can be shown that when an inert gas dissolved in saline in steadily infused into the venous circulation, the proportion of the gas which is eliminated by ventilation from the blood of a given alveolus depends on its ventilation-perfusion ratio [7]. Furthermore, the higher the solubility of the gas, the smaller is the proportion eliminated at a given ventilation-perfusion ratio. Thus while almost all of an almost insoluble gas like helium is eliminated by alveoli even when their ventilation-perfusion ratio is as low as 0.1, little of a very soluble gas like ethyl ether is eliminated by alveoli when their ventilation-perfusion ratio is as high as 10. By using a mixture of gases of different solubilities and measuring their elimination rates, it might therefore be possible to determine the proportions of the lung having alveoli of known ventilation-perfusion ratios. This would approach one of the goals of the respiratory physiologist which is to draw a frequency distribution of ventilation-perfusion ratios in the abnormal lung. An interesting feature of the inert gas technique is that an attempt is being made to unravel the problems of gas exchange without using the natural respiratory gases. Indeed from the physiologist's point of view, the chief convenience of these gases is that they are there; it may well be that foreign gases have more useful properties for the measurement of ventilation-perfusion ratio inequality.

How to differentiate ventilation-perfusion ratio inequality from other causes of hypoxaemia

Chapter 1 was devoted to the four causes of arterial hypoxaemia: hypoventilation, impaired diffusion, true shunt and ventilation-perfusion ratio inequality. The first can be looked upon as an exaggeration of the normal fall in P_{O_2} which occurs when air is inspired into the alveoli, whereas the last three causes can be considered as imperfections of the actual lung because they each cause an alveolar-arterial difference for P_{O_2}. This is small in the normal lung but may become large in the diseased lung. How can we separate these four causes of arterial hypoxaemia?

Effect of breathing pure oxygen

By giving a patient pure oxygen to breathe, true shunt can be distinguished from the other causes of hypoxaemia because only in this condition does hypoxaemia remain. True shunt (figure 7) here means all the blood which finds its way into the arterial blood without going through ventilated lung. This includes right-to-left intracardiac shunts, abnormal communications between the pulmonary arteries and veins within the lung, and alveoli which are perfused but completely unventilated. It might be argued that the last should be included under the heading of ventilation-perfusion ratio inequality rather than true shunt since these alveoli are simply at the bottom end of the ventilation-perfusion ratio line (figures 23 and 24) with a ratio of nil. It is more convenient however to regard these unventilated alveoli as true shunt because their effects on gas exchange are undistinguishable from those of the other shunts.

It is easy to see how breathing pure oxygen abolishes the hypoxaemia of hypoventilation, diffusion impairment and ventilation-perfusion ratio inequality. Suppose extreme hypoventilation reduced the alveolar P_{O_2} to 20 mmHg while the P_{CO_2} rose to 108 mmHg, these figures being obtained by moving the alveolar point along the gas R line of 0.8 (figure 31). On pure oxygen, the nitrogen would be washed out and the alveolar P_{O_2} would be atmospheric pressure less P_{CO_2} less P_{H_2O} or $760 - 108 - 47 = 605$ mmHg. This is some six times the normal alveolar P_{O_2} when

the lung is breathing air and emphasises what a powerful physiological tool is pure oxygen. A similar argument applies in the case
of ventilation-perfusion ratio inequality. Suppose alveoli with
a very low ventilation-perfusion ratio had an alveolar P_{O_2} of
50 mmHg and an alveolar P_{CO_2} of 45 mmHg, these figures being
obtained by moving the alveolar point along the ventilation-
perfusion ratio line (figure 24). Again when the nitrogen is washed
out by pure oxygen, the alveolar P_{O_2} would be $760 - 45 - 47 =$
668 mmHg. Indeed a moment's thought will show that the
ventilation-perfusion ratio line when the lung breathes pure oxygen is straight with a slope of minus one because as the ventilation-
perfusion ratio is reduced and the P_{CO_2} rises, the P_{O_2} will fall at the
same rate (figure 50). It is true that it might take many minutes

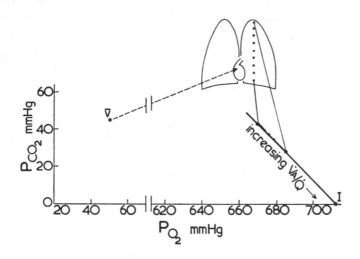

Figure 50. Oxygen-carbon dioxide diagram for the normal lung breathing
pure oxygen. Note that the horizontal axis has been broken and is in fact
very elongated. The ventilation-perfusion ratio line is straight with a slope
of -1 because the sum of $P_{O_2} + P_{CO_2}$ is constant (being equal to $P_B -$
P_{H_2O}). No matter how low the ventilation-perfusion ratio (as long as it is
above zero), the alveolar P_{O_2} is high. However unventilated alveoli have a
P_{O_2} of about 50 mm Hg. Thus breathing pure oxygen differentiates
between hypoxaemia caused by ventilation-perfusion ratio inequality and
hypoxaemia caused by unventilated alveoli.

for the nitrogen to be washed out if these alveoli are very poorly ventilated but as long as they are ventilated, alveolar P_{O_2} is bound to rise greatly. Finally in a lung with impaired diffusion, any hypoxaemia breathing air is relieved by oxygen because this so enormously increases the driving pressure moving oxygen across the blood-gas barrier. Figure 5A shows that a corpuscle entering the pulmonary capillary is normally exposed to a P_{O_2} difference of about 60 mmHg between itself and the alveolar gas. When the lung breathes oxygen, this driving pressure is increased to some 600 mmHg and this ten-fold increase is ample to force the oxygen across.

It should be noted that in a patient with a true shunt, the arterial P_{O_2} will rise appreciably when pure oxygen is breathed. This is because the unshunted blood which passes through ventilated alveoli picks up more dissolved oxygen (although the haemoglobin is normally nearly 100% saturated). This extra oxygen may raise the arterial oxygen saturation from 75% to very nearly 100% but a measurement of arterial P_{O_2} will always allow the amount of shunt to be calculated.

Effect of breathing a low oxygen mixture

Low oxygen mixtures are of little value in differentiating between the four causes of arterial hypoxaemia. In each instance, the hypoxaemia becomes more severe and indeed the procedure may cause dangerously low levels of arterial P_{O_2} if care is not taken. The manoeuvre is mentioned here because at one time it was thought that by using a low oxygen mixture, it was possible to distinguish between diffusion impairment and ventilation-perfusion ratio inequality. The basis for this belief was that a low alveolar P_{O_2} exaggerates diffusion difficulties (figure 5B) whereas the effect of a true shunt on the arterial P_{O_2} is small when the alveolar P_{O_2} is low. This is because the effect of shunted blood is to reduce the arterial oxygen *content* by a defined amount, and the consequent lowering of P_{O_2} is smaller when the arterial P_{O_2} is initially low and the slope of the oxygen dissociation curve is steep (figure 27A). Thus if venous admixture behaved like a true shunt when a low oxygen mixture was breathed, ventilation-perfusion ratio inequality would result in a small P_{O_2} difference between ideal alveolar gas and arterial blood (figure 40), whereas diffusion impairment would make this difference large.

More recently, it has been appreciated that although venous admixture behaves like a true shunt in one respect in that both depress the arterial P_{O_2}, the analogy does not extend to the effect of alveolar hypoxia on the arterial P_{O_2}. In fact, calculations show that far from the venous admixture effect always becoming small when a low oxygen mixture is breathed, it may become large. The behaviour of the arterial P_{O_2} during alveolar hypoxia is determined in a complicated way by the pattern of uneven ventilation and blood flow. Thus the 'two level oxygen method' for measuring diffusing capacity is now little used.

Association of raised arterial P_{CO_2}

The arterial P_{CO_2} is of value in distinguishing between the four causes of arterial hypoxaemia. Hypoventilation is *always* accompanied by a raised arterial P_{CO_2} because it interferes with the elimination of carbon dioxide as much as with the uptake of oxygen. The relation between the arterial P_{O_2} and P_{CO_2} during hypoventilation can be predicted from the oxygen-carbon dioxide diagram because the alveolar and arterial points (neglecting for a moment the normal small alveolar-arterial difference) will move up the appropriate gas R line (figure 51). The particular R is fixed by the metabolic demands of the whole body. Notice that this implies considerable carbon dioxide retention at only moderate degrees of hypoxia; thus figure 51 shows that at an R of 0.8, the arterial P_{CO_2} is as high as 80 mmHg when the alveolar P_{O_2} is only reduced to 45 mmHg. Although the arterial P_{O_2} will be a few mmHg lower than this, the arterial oxygen saturation will probably be above 75% and cyanosis may not be detectable. Thus carbon dioxide retention is usually more of a problem than hypoxaemia. This is particularly the case if the patient is breathing an oxygen enriched mixture when dangerous hypercarbia may be present in spite of a 'healthy' pink colour.

Impaired diffusion tends to be associated with a low arterial P_{CO_2} because carbon dioxide diffusion is rapid and little affected

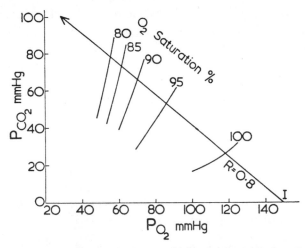

Figure 51. Blood gas changes during hypoventilation. In this figure, the alveolar-arterial differences have been neglected so that both alveolar and arterial points rise along the gas R line. Note that the arterial P_{CO_2} rises to about 80 mmHg before the oxygen saturation falls below 75% and cyanosis can be detected with reasonable certainty. The effect of any alveolar-arterial difference would be to lower the arterial P_{O_2} further.

by any thickening of the alveolar membrane, and ventilation is often increased by the additional hypoxic drive. The arterial P_{CO_2} in patients with true shunts is usually normal because large portions of the lung are unaffected and capable of eliminating carbon dioxide in response to the ventilatory drive from the respiratory centre. The arterial P_{CO_2} accompanying ventilation-perfusion ratio inequality may be high, normal or low. The development of carbon dioxide retention in this condition was discussed on page 81.

Effect of exercise

This is of limited value in distinguishing between the causes of hypoxaemia. In hypoventilation, hypoxaemia typically becomes more severe on exercise because the oxygen uptake is increased and the lung responds sluggishly to the added ventilatory drive. The patient with impaired diffusion usually becomes more cyanosed on exercise because an increased oxygen uptake is an additional stress to the diffusion process (figure 5) resulting in a larger P_{O_2} difference between alveolar gas and end-capillary blood. A true shunt which remains a constant proportion of the cardiac output on exercise causes more hypoxaemia because the P_{O_2} of the mixed venous blood and therefore of the shunted blood is lower. Finally the hypoxaemia of a patient with ventilation-perfusion ratio inequality may become worse or improve depending on his ventilatory response and the pattern of uneven distribution in the lung.

How to talk the $\dot{V}A/\dot{Q}$ language

Symbols have been omitted from the main text of this monograph because initially most people are discouraged by them. However some kind of shorthand is essential if the quantities are to be manipulated algebraically. Fortunately there is now very wide agreement on most of the symbols used [19].

General

V	Gas volume
$\dot{V}$	Gas volume per unit time
P	Gas pressure
F	Fractional concentration of gas in dry phase
R	Respiratory exchange ratio i.e. $\dot{V}_{CO_2}/\dot{V}_{O_2}$
Q	Volume flow of blood
C	Concentration in blood phase

Gas phase only

I	Inspired gas
E	Expired gas
A	Alveolar gas
B	Barometric
D	Dead space gas

Blood phase only

a	Arterial
v	Venous
$\bar{v}$	Mixed venous

These symbols for blood and gas are used as subscripts.

To demonstrate the use of these symbols, two key equations are derived below.

Ventilation-perfusion ratio equation

The amount of CO_2 lost from alveolar gas per minute is given by

$$\dot{V}_{CO_2} = \dot{V}_A.P_{A CO_2}.K$$

where the inspired gas contains no CO_2, $\dot{V}_A$ means expired alveolar ventilation, and K is a constant.

The amount of CO_2 lost from capillary blood per minute is given by

$$\dot{V}_{CO_2} = \dot{Q}(C\bar{v}_{CO_2} - Ca_{CO_2}) \quad \text{(Fick equation)}$$

In a steady state, these must be the same. Thus

$$\dot{V}_A.P_{A CO_2}.K = \dot{Q}(C\bar{v}_{CO_2} - Ca_{CO_2})$$

or

$$\dot{V}_A/\dot{Q} = \frac{C\bar{v}_{CO_2} - Ca_{CO_2}}{P_{A CO_2}.K} \qquad (1)$$

Since Ca_{CO_2} and $P_{A CO_2}$ are linked by the CO_2 dissociation curve (assuming complete equilibration for CO_2 along the pulmonary capillary, figure 5), this equation means that if the inspired gas contains no CO_2, the alveolar and arterial P_{CO_2} are uniquely determined by the CO_2 content of mixed venous blood and the ventilation-perfusion ratio. Thus we have proved what was assumed intuitively on page 35. Analogous equations can be written down for O_2.

When the body temperature is $37°C$, $\dot{V}_A$ is in litres/min B.T.P.S., and the contents are in ml of gas S.T.P.D./100 ml blood, K has the value $1/8.63$. Thus the equation is often written

$$\dot{V}_A/\dot{Q} = \frac{8.63\ (C\bar{v}_{CO_2} - Ca_{CO_2})}{P_{A.CO_2}}$$

Alveolar gas equation

This is the equation by which the ideal alveolar P_{O_2} is calculated knowing the composition of inspired gas, R, and the ideal alveolar P_{CO_2} (assumed equal to the arterial P_{CO_2}, see page 92 and figure 47).

R is given by $\quad \dfrac{\dot{V}_{CO_2}}{\dot{V}_{O_2}}$

Now $\dot{V}_{CO_2} = \dot{V}_{AE}.F_{ACO_2}$ (no CO_2 in inspired gas)
and $\dot{V}_{O_2} = (\dot{V}_{AI}.F_{IO_2} - \dot{V}_{AE}.F_{AO_2})$

where $\dot{V}_{AI}$ and $\dot{V}_{AE}$ are inspired and expired alveolar ventilations respectively.

Thus

$$R = \frac{\dot{V}_{AE}.F_{ACO_2}}{\dot{V}_{AI}.F_{IO_2} - \dot{V}_{AE}.F_{AO_2}}$$

$$= \frac{F_{ACO_2}}{F_{IO_2}.\dfrac{\dot{V}_{AI}}{\dot{V}_{AE}} - F_{AO_2}} \qquad (2)$$

To find the ratio of inspired to expired alveolar ventilation, we can use the fact that the quantities of nitrogen inspired and expired are the same. Since $F_{O_2} + F_{CO_2} + F_{N_2} = 1$, the quantity of N_2 entering the alveoli each minute is $\dot{V}_{AI}(1 - F_{IO_2} - F_{ICO_2})$ and the quantity leaving is $\dot{V}_{AE}(1 - F_{AO_2} - F_{ACO_2})$. Thus $\dot{V}_{AI}(1 - F_{IO_2} - F_{ICO_2}) = \dot{V}_{AE}(1 - F_{AO_2} - F_{ACO_2})$ and since F_{ICO_2} is negligible when the patient breaths air,

$$\frac{\dot{V}_{AI}}{\dot{V}_{AE}} = \frac{1 - F_{AO_2} - F_{ACO_2}}{1 - F_{IO_2}}$$

Thus equation 2 becomes

$$R = \frac{F_{ACO_2}}{F_{IO_2} \dfrac{1 - F_{AO_2} - F_{ACO_2}}{1 - F_{IO_2}} - F_{AO_2}}$$

From which $F_{AO_2} = F_{IO_2} - \dfrac{F_{ACO_2}}{R} + F_{ACO_2}.F_{IO_2}.\dfrac{(1-R)}{R}$

Since fractional concentration and partial pressure are related by the expression $P_x = F_x(P_B - 47)$ where $P_{H_2O} = 47$ mmHg, we may write

$$P_{AO_2} = P_{IO_2} - \frac{P_{ACO_2}}{R} + P_{ACO_2}.F_{IO_2}.\frac{(1-R)}{R} \qquad (3)$$

which is the alveolar gas equation. (See page 92.)

How to draw a $\dot{V}A/\dot{Q}$ line

To become familiar with the O_2-CO_2 diagram, the serious reader should draw a $\dot{V}A/\dot{Q}$ line. This is conveniently done on chart I at the back of '*A Graphical Analysis of the Respiratory Gas Exchange*' by Rahn and Fenn [21] or on a thin sheet of graph paper laid over this (Chartwell no. 5205 bank paper is suitable).

First mark the inspired gas point ($P_{O_2} = 149$ mmHg; $P_{CO_2} = 0$) and choose a mixed venous point (say $P_{O_2} = 40$ mmHg; $P_{CO_2} = 45$ mmHg). Next draw the gas R lines (figure 30) either by using the transparent overlay provided or more accurately, by calculating the $P_{A_{O_2}}$ for a $P_{A_{CO_2}}$ of 60 mmHg and various values of R using the alveolar gas equation. Mark these points on the diagram and join them to the inspired point. Now trace in the O_2 and CO_2 content isopleths (figure 28) noting that the O_2 lines do not take dissolved O_2 into account so that some inaccuracy occurs at high P_{O_2}.

We are now ready to construct the $\dot{V}A/\dot{Q}$ line. Originally this was done by drawing the blood R lines and noting their points of intersection with the appropriate gas R lines (figure 31). Essentially the same answer is given by a faster trial and error technique. In the equation

$$C\bar{v}_{CO_2} - R(Ca_{O_2} - C\bar{v}_{O_2}) = Ca_{CO_2}$$

we know $C\bar{v}_{CO_2}$ and $C\bar{v}_{O_2}$. The technique consists of choosing a value of R and then finding values of Ca_{O_2} and Ca_{CO_2} by trial and error which satisfy the equation. Thus when $C\bar{v}_{CO_2} = 52.4$ vols % and $C\bar{v}_{O_2} = 14.6$ vols % and $R = 0.8$, it is found by moving up and down the $R = 0.8$ line that the equation is only satisfied when $Ca_{O_2} = 19.55$ and $Ca_{CO_2} = 48.4$ vols %. In practice, this procedure is rapid and can be accomplished for a dozen R values in a few minutes. The $\dot{V}_A/\dot{Q}$ line is then drawn by joining the individual points.

The value of $\dot{V}_A/\dot{Q}$ at various points along the line is found from the ventilation-perfusion ratio equation

$$\dot{V}_A/\dot{Q} = 8.63 \frac{(C\bar{v}_{CO_2} - Ca_{CO_2})}{P_{ACO_2}}$$

where the contents are in vols/100 vols.

When this has been done, it is possible to plot P_{AO_2}, P_{ACO_2}, P_{AN_2} and R against $\dot{V}_A/\dot{Q}$ and to calculate the gas exchange in various lung models. The reader may like to check the calculations shown in figures 26, 29 and 35. These calculations were made using a $\dot{V}_A/\dot{Q}$ line drawn for $P\bar{v}_{O_2} = 40$ and $P\bar{v}_{CO_2} = 45$ mmHg and some of the values are shown in table 1. Small deviations from these should not be considered important because of the uncertainties in the O_2 and CO_2 dissociation curves.

Table I. Calculated values from the $\dot{V}_A/\dot{Q}$ line for mixed venous blood of $P_{O_2} = 40$, $P_{CO_2} = 45$ mmHg, and inspired gas $P_{O_2} = 149$ mm Hg and $P_{CO_2} = 0$

R	$\dot{V}_A/\dot{Q}$	P_{O_2} mmHg	P_{CO_2} mmHg	C_{O_2} vols %	C_{CO_2} vols %
0.357	0	40.0	45.0	14.6	52.4
0.4	0.16	51.5	44.5	16.6	51.6
0.45	0.30	62.4	44.0	18.0	50.9
0.5	0.38	70.6	43.7	18.5	50.5
0.6	0.55	84.2	42.4	19.0	49.7
0.7	0.70	93.8	41.3	19.4	49.0
0.8	0.86	100.8	40.0	19.55	48.4
0.9	1.01	106.8	39.0	19.65	47.9
1.0	1.18	111.3	37.7	19.75	47.2
1.2	1.56	118.2	35.2	19.90	46.0
1.5	2.15	124.9	32.5	20.0	44.3
2.0	3.34	132.2	27.9	20.0	41.6
3.0	7.0	139.5	20.0	20.0	36.2

Recently, computer programmes for drawing $\dot{V}_A/\dot{Q}$ lines have been developed [12, 18]. These allow the solution of problems of gas exchange which previously were impossibly complicated [26].

Suggestions for further reading

This list includes some of the early papers on ventilation-perfusion inequality and a few more recent articles.

BRISCOE W.A. & COURNAND A. (1962) The degree of variation of blood perfusion and of ventilation within the emphysematous lung, and some related considerations. In: *Pulmonary Structure and Function*, ed. by A.V.S. de Reuck and M. O'Connor. J. & A. Churchill, Ltd.

COMROE J.H., Jr., FORSTER R.E. (II), DUBOIS A.B., BRISCOE W.A. & CARLSEN, ELIZABETH (1962) *'The Lung'*, Second Edition. Year Book Medical Publishers, Chicago.

DONALD K.W., RENZETTI A., RILEY R.L. & COURNAND A. (1952) Analysis of factors affecting concentration of oxygen and carbon dioxide in gas and blood of lungs: results. *J. Appl. Physiol.* **4**, 497–525.

FARHI L.E. (1966) Ventilation-perfusion relationship and its role in alveolar gas exchange. In: *'Advances in Respiratory Physiology'*. ed. by C. Caro. W.H. Arnold, London.

FARHI L.E. & RAHN H. (1955) A theoretical analysis of the alveolar-arterial O_2 difference with special reference to the distribution effect. *J. Appl. Physiol.* **7**, 699–703.

FENN W.O., RAHN H. & OTIS A.B. (1946) A theoretical study of the composition of alveolar air at altitude. *Amer. J. Physiol.* **146**, 637–653.

RAHN H. (1949) A concept of mean alveolar air and the ventilation-blood flow relationships during pulmonary gas exchange. *Amer. J. Physiol.* **158**, 21–30.

RAHN H. & FARHI L.E. (1962) Ventilation-perfusion relationship. In: *Pulmonary Structure and Function*. ed. by A.V.S. de Reuck and M. O'Connor. J. & A. Churchill, Ltd.

RAHN H. & FARHI L.E. (1964) Ventilation, perfusion, and gas exchange—the $\dot{V}_A/\dot{Q}$ concept. In: *Handbook of Physiology*. Section 3, vol. 1, 735–765. ed. by W.O. Fenn and H. Rahn. Amer. Physiol. Soc., Washington.

RAHN H. & FENN W.O. (1956) *A Graphical Analysis of the Respiratory Gas Exchange*. The Amer. Physiol. Soc., Washington, D.C.

READ J. & FOWLER K.T. (1962) The non-homogeneous lung. *Aust. Annals Med.* **11**, 129–143.

RILEY R.L. & COURNAND A. (1949) 'Ideal' alveolar air and the analysis of ventilation-perfusion relationships in the lungs. *J. Appl. Physiol.* **1**, 825–847.

RILEY R.L. & COURNAND A. (1951) Analysis of factors affecting partial pressures of oxygen and carbon dioxide in gas and blood of lungs: theory. *J. Appl. Physiol.* **4**, 77–101.

RILEY R.L., COURNAND A. & DONALD K.W. (1951) Analysis of factors affecting partial pressures of oxygen and carbon dioxide in gas and blood of lungs: methods. *J. Appl. Physiol.* **4**, 102–120.

References

This is not intended to be a comprehensive list. These papers have been cited in the text either because the points are disputed or because the work is relatively recent or not well known.

[1] BEVEGARD S., HOLMGREN A. & JONSSON B. (1960) The effect of body position on the circulation at rest and during exercise, with special reference to the influence on the stroke volume. *Acta Physiol. Scand.* **49**, 279–298.

[2] BRISCOE W.A. (1959) A method for dealing with data concerning uneven ventilation of the lung and its effects on blood gas transfer. *J. Appl. Physiol.* **14**, 291–298.

[3] BRYAN A.C., BENTIVOGLIO L.G., BEEREL F., MACLEISH H., ZIDULKA A. & BATES D.V. (1964) Factors affecting regional distribution of ventilation and perfusion in the lung. *J. Appl. Physiol.* **19**, 395–402.

[4] CANFIELD R.E. & RAHN H. (1957) Arterial-alveolar N_2 gas pressure differences due to ventilation-perfusion variations. *J. Appl. Physiol.* **10**, 165–172.

[5] COLE R.B. & BISHOP J.M. (1963) Effect of varying inspired O_2 tension on alveolar-arterial O_2 tension differences in man. *J. Appl. Physiol.* **18**, 1043–1048.

[6] DONALD K.W., RENZETTI A., RILEY R.L. & COURNAND A. (1952) Analysis of factors affecting concentrations of oxygen and carbon dioxide in gas and blood of lungs: results. *J. Appl. Physiol.* **4**, 497–525.

[7] FAHRI L.E. (1967) Elimination of inert gas by the lung. *Respir. Physiol.* **3** 1–11.

[8] FINLEY T.N., SWENSON E.W. & COMROE J.H. (1962) The cause of arterial hypoxaemia at rest in patients with 'alveolar-capillary block syndrome'. *J. Clin. Invest.* **41**, 618–622.

[9] GLAZIER J.B., HUGHES J.M.B., MALONEY J.E. & WEST J.B. (1967) Vertical gradient of alveolar size in lungs of dogs frozen intact. *J. Appl. Physiol.* **23**, 694–705.

[10] GLAZIER J.B., HUGHES J.M.B., MALONEY J.E. & WEST J.B. (1969) Measurements of capillary dimensions and blood volume in rapidly frozen lungs. *J. Appl. Physiol.* **26**, 65–76.

[11] HUGHES J.M.B., GLAZIER J.B., MALONEY J.E. & WEST J.B. (1968) Effect of lung volume on the distribution of pulmonary blood flow in man. *Respir. Physiol.* **4**, 58–72.

[12] KELMAN G.R. (1968) Computer program for the production of O_2-CO_2 diagrams. *Respir. Physiol.* **4**, 260–269.

[13] KLOCKE F.J. & RAHN H. (1961) The arterial-alveolar inert gas ('N_2') difference in normal and emphysematous subjects, as indicated by the analysis of urine. *J. Clin. Invest.* **40**, 286–294.

[14] LENFANT C. (1963) Measurement of ventilation-perfusion distribution with alveolar-arterial differences. *J. Appl. Physiol.* **18**, 1090–1094.

[15] MALONEY J.E., BERGEL D.H., GLAZIER J.B., HUGHES J.M.B. & WEST J.B. (1968) Effect of pulsatile pulmonary artery pressure on distribution of blood flow in isolated lung. *Respir. Physiol.* **4**, 154–167.

[16] MALONEY J.E., BERGEL D.H., GLAZIER J.B., HUGHES J.M.B. & WEST J.B. (1968) Transmission of pulsatile blood pressure and flow through the isolated lung. *Circ. Res.*, **23**, 11–24.

[17] MILIC-EMILI J., HENDERSON J.A.M., DOLOVICH M.B., TROP D. & KANEKO P. (1966) Regional distribution of inspired gas in the lung. *J. Appl. Physiol.* **21**, 749–759.

[18] OLSZOWKA A.J. & FARHI L.E. (1969) A digital computer program for constructing ventilation-perfusion lines. *J. Appl. Physiol.* **26**, 141–146.

[19] PAPPENHEIMER J. (1950) Standardization of definitions and symbols in respiratory physiology. *Fed. Proc.* **9**, 602–605.

[20] PERMUTT S. (1965) Effect of interstitial pressure of the lung on pulmonary circulation. *Med. thorac.* **22**, 118–131.

[21] RAHN H. & FENN W.O. (1956) *A Graphical Analysis of the Respiratory Gas Exchange.* The Amer. Physiol. Soc., Washington, D.C.

[22] READ J. & WILLIAMS R.S. (1959) Pulmonary ventilation/blood flow relationships in interstitial disease of the lungs. *Amer. J. Med.* **27**, 545–550.

[23] RILEY R.L. & COURNAND A. (1949) 'Ideal' alveolar air and the analysis of ventilation-perfusion relationships in the lungs. *J. Appl. Physiol.* **1**, 825–847.

[24] RILEY R.L. & COURNAND A. (1951) Analysis of factors affecting partial pressures of oxygen and carbon dioxide in gas and blood of lungs: theory. *J. Appl. Physiol.* **4**, 77–101.

[25] RILEY R.L., COURNAND A. & DONALD K.W. (1951) Analysis of factors affecting partial pressures of oxygen and carbon dioxide in gas and blood of lungs: methods. *J. Appl. Physiol.* **4**, 102–120.

[26] WEST J.B. (1969) Ventilation-perfusion inequality and overall gas exchange in computer models of the lung. *Respir. Physiol.* **7**, 88–110.

[27] WEST J.B., FOWLER K.T., HUGH-JONES P. & O'DONNELL T.V. (1957) Measurement of the ventilation-perfusion ratio inequality in the lung by the analysis of a single expirate. *Clin. Sci.* **16**, 529–547.

[28] WEST J.B., FOWLER K.T., HUGH-JONES P. & O'DONNELL T.V. (1957) The measurement of the inequality of ventilation and of perfusion in the lung by the analysis of single expirates. *Clin. Sci.* **16**, 549–565.

Index